# Just One
## of the Kids

## Raising a Resilient Family
## When One of Your Children
## Has a Physical Disability

KAY HARRIS KRIEGSMAN, Ph.D., and
SARA PALMER, Ph.D.

The Johns Hopkins University Press

*Baltimore*

© 2013 Kay Harris Kriegsman and Sara Palmer
All rights reserved. Published 2013
Printed in the United States of America on acid-free paper
9  8  7  6  5  4  3  2  1

The Johns Hopkins University Press
2715 North Charles Street
Baltimore, Maryland 21218-4363
www.press.jhu.edu

Library of Congress Cataloging-in-Publication Data

Kriegsman, Kay Harris.
    Just one of the kids : raising a resilient family when one of your children has a physical disability / Kay Harris Kriegsman, Ph.D., and Sara Palmer, Ph.D.
        pages cm
    Includes bibliographical references and index.
    ISBN 978-1-4214-0930-6 (hardcover : alk. paper) — ISBN 1-4214-0930-5 (hardcover : alk. paper) — ISBN 978-1-4214-0931-3 (pbk. : alk. paper) — ISBN 1-4214-0931-3 (pbk. : alk. paper) — ISBN 978-1-4214-0932-0 (electronic) — ISBN 1-4214-0932-1 (electronic)
    1. Children with disabilities—Family relationships.  2. Parents of children with disabilities. I. Palmer, Sara.  II. Title.
    HQ773.6.K75 2013
    649′.151—dc23        2012035771

A catalog record for this book is available from the British Library.

*Special discounts are available for bulk purchases of this book. For more information, please contact Special Sales at 410-516-6936 or specialsales@press.jhu.edu.*

The Johns Hopkins University Press uses environmentally friendly book materials, including recycled text paper that is composed of at least 30 percent post-consumer waste, whenever possible.

This book is dedicated to you, the families hailing from Vancouver to Massachusetts, Wisconsin to South Carolina, whose stories form the backbone of this book. Mothers and fathers, grandmothers and grandfathers, and brothers and sisters, both able-bodied and with physical disabilities, you talked with us face-to-face, by telephone, or via e-mail. You generously shared details of your emotional and family lives, describing the day-to-day challenges and rewards of being a family that includes a child who has a physical disability. You inspired us with your hopefulness and creativity in developing what you needed to forge ahead. This book could not have been written without you.

# Contents

----------------------------------------------------------------------------

## Part III: Into the Wide World

## Why This Book?

Where do you go for information, encouragement, and advice when you have a child who has a physical disability? In our work with children and adults who have physical disabilities and with their parents and families, we discovered that there are many books and articles for parents raising children with cognitive or emotional disabilities. Few, however, address the needs of families that include a child who has a *physical* disability but is cognitively normal and emotionally healthy. The challenges these kids face overlap to some extent with the challenges of kids who have cognitive disabilities, but these children also have distinctly different challenges—and different capabilities. People who have *physical* disabilities have the mental and emotional capability to engage independently in adult activities, although they may need physical help to do so. People who have cognitive or emotional disabilities may not need physical help but may depend on parents (or others) for cognitive and emotional assistance on into adulthood.

At small local meetings, at national conferences on physical disability, and in our clinical practices, families of children who have a physical disability have expressed their need for information to help them raise their children successfully. They wanted guidance on how to create more inclusive families, in which each of their kids, whether or not they have disabilities, would be able to participate in social life, recreation, and education and be prepared for employment or other productive activities in adulthood. And they wanted to know how to access opportunities and resources, within and outside the family, to make this possible.

Our book aims to help parents and children achieve these goals. It is written specifically for and about parents of families that include a child who has a physical disability and one or more children who are able-bodied—mostly from the perspective of real parents, who volunteered to share their experiences with us. (One family whose story is featured in the book has a son who has a physical disability and no other children.) In writing this book, we did extensive interviews not only with the parents but also with grandparents and children, both able-bodied and with physical disabilities, from many families. We sifted through their experiences to identify the tools they developed and used, as well as the ones they were searching for in their quest to raise healthy, happy children prepared for successful adulthood. This book combines the wisdom of these families with our own personal and professional experience and the work of other disability experts to present a framework for raising resilient children. Included are many tips, tools, suggestions, and resources to help you raise *your* family. (Look for the ⚠, ☞, and ⊤ symbols throughout.)

The names of all people we interviewed have been changed to protect their privacy, and all names used in the family stories or elsewhere in the book are pseudonyms. Some people portrayed are composites of multiple people.

## Why Us? Personal Perspectives

Kay always wondered as a child, "What's the big deal about having a physical disability?" She did the same things her brothers did, albeit from a sitting stance or using crutches and braces, after a bout with polio at age 7. They all played musical instruments, were active in 4-H, did assigned chores, helped care for two younger sisters born many years later, had the usual childhood fights, and bottle-fed the "bummer lambs," abandoned at birth by their mothers.

Although she had physical therapy, operations, and doctors' appointments, Kay was also just one of the kids and felt included and needed in the larger family scene. Disability was just one of a number of challenges her family faced, the chief one being economic upheaval, at times requiring both of her parents to work outside the home. While this was hard on the family, it had a positive side for Kay, as it took the focus off her disability and meant that she had to be a contributing member of the family. She washed dishes, set the table, and vacuumed while sitting on the floor.

Kay was not aware as a child how her disability affected her parents. While her family treated her like any other child, it wasn't always easy. Kay's mother still remembers that just after her daughter was airlifted from their small mountain town to a big-city hospital, the head of the hospital billing office was disdainful and made her feel incompetent because their family had no health insurance. Kay's brothers felt the effects of their sister's eight-month hospitalization. Like other children during the polio epidemics, in the first few weeks of Kay's illness her brothers were quarantined. They were angry with the landlord, who demanded the rent when their mother returned home from taking Kay to the distant hospital, so they showed the landlord what they thought of him, taking a knife and "decorating" the woodwork in the house. Their mother laughed and cried with pride in her sons' misguided protection of her, while wondering how she could ever pay for the repair.

When Kay returned home from the coddled atmosphere of the hospital, her family had new responsibilities to shoulder. Getting on with life meant adding new activities; for instance, Kay's mother had to do physical therapy exercises with her every day.

In the years following, Kay never heard from her family that she could *not* do something. If there were a student council meeting on the second floor of a building without an elevator, her family would find a way for her to attend; usually, her brothers "bumped" her up the steps in her wheelchair. It was expected that she would ask a boy to the Sadie Hawkins Day dance, go on 4-H trips, and drive a car at age 16. Although her family encouraged her to take risks, there were times when they weren't comfortable with what Kay herself was ready to do. Although Kay walked with crutches except through her high school's busy hallways (where she used a wheelchair), her family assumed that she would take her wheelchair to college for safety and to conserve her energy—and use it. She refused. The compromise was that the wheelchair took the ride over the Continental Divide to the university and then was safely stowed away in the basement of the dorm.

Kay's parents made a choice to see what *could be* rather than what *could have been*. Her parents must have been saddened when their little 7-year-old girl, who loved dancing and "running the hills" with her brothers, had to begin using double leg braces and crutches to walk. But they never conveyed a sense that they saw her as anything but an equal to her brothers and sisters, neither less nor more. They always chose to deal with "what is."

The acceptance and equal treatment by her family shaped Kay's attitudes about physical disability and her interest in helping other families raise hearty, independent-minded kids—whether or not they have a physical disability. You will see many of her experiences echoed in the stories of other families we interviewed for this book.

With the love and support of Will, her late husband, Kay returned to graduate school to work on her PhD in counseling while mothering Bill and Katie. For many years she codirected the HOW (Handicapped Is Only a Word) Conference, an annual event for teenagers who have physical disabilities, their parents, and their teen siblings. HOW emphasized opportunities for socialization, peer support, future planning, and fun. Kay's work with families—parents, children who have disabilities and their siblings, and some grandparents, as well—expanded from one-on-one sessions to small groups to large conventions. She published a book for teenagers who have physical disabilities, coauthored two books with Sara, and published articles on disability in professional journals and consumer magazines. She maintains a private psychology practice working with people, both able-bodied and who have disabilities, going through the normal ups and downs of life.

Sara grew up able-bodied in a family that was not directly affected by physical disability. Much of her experience with disability has come from her work as a rehabilitation psychologist, helping people who have disabilities and their partners and families cope with difficult circumstances and live more fulfilling lives.

Sara's course work for her PhD in clinical psychology included nothing about physical disability. But her husband was in medical school at the time, and he planned to specialize in physical medicine and rehabilitation. Through him, Sara was introduced to the field of rehabilitation psychology, met more people who had disabilities, and was inspired to explore this new career path. During her internship at the Seattle VA Hospital, Sara elected to spend three months on the inpatient rehabilitation unit, evaluating and treating people with spinal cord injuries, strokes, amputations, multiple sclerosis, and other disabilities. She found it refreshing to work with people who were generally mentally healthy but were coping with the emotional fallout from a life-changing accident or illness. Colleagues often asked her if it was depressing to work with people who had such "tragic" circumstances, but Sara felt uplifted by the strength and creativity she saw in her patients as they discovered ways to cope with their disabilities and reengage in life. She signed on for another three-month elective, and rehabilitation psychology has been the focus of her career ever since.

Over the years, Sara has worked in various hospitals and in private practice. She has worked with many teens and young adults who have disabilities and with their families, in addition to adults and seniors. She has written books about spinal cord injury and stroke for people who have these conditions and for their families. She has volunteered with disability organizations and been an educator and advocate within her profession for people who have disabilities. Sara has learned an enormous amount about living with a physical disability from her friendship and professional collaboration with Kay, spanning more than twenty-five years.

We hope this book will urge you on to claim the excitement and possibilities that exist in you and your family, finding the "aha" moment as you transition from feeling the "*burden*" of disability to the joy of *discovery*, when you begin to think, "What if we try it *this* way?"

## In Appreciation

We have many to thank, beginning with Jackie Wehmueller, the most gracious, instructive, and supportive of editors, who guided us through two earlier books and helped us hone our voice in this one. Our appreciation for her wise counsel, soothing voice, honesty, and concern cannot be adequately put into words.

We thank Jeremy Horsefield, whose copyediting further improved the tone and readability of the manuscript.

We are grateful to Armetta Parker of United Cerebral Palsy, Charleene Frazier of the Spinal Cord Injury Network, Kevin Fang, Sherry Arvin of the Spina Bifida Association, the staff of the Osteogenesis Imperfecta Foundation, and the staff of the Arthritis Foundation, who put out the call to parents, siblings, and grandparents who wanted to be interviewed for the book. Their assistance was invaluable.

Finally, we thank our families, who are always there for us: Kay's mother, Elizabeth Harris; her siblings, John, Dick, Beth, and Sue Harris; and her children and grandchildren, Bill, Christy, and Kyle Kriegsman, and Katie, Jerry, Darby, Raymond, and Addy Peters; Sara's father, Irving Sarnoff; her brother, David Pepper Sarnoff, and his wife, Pepper Sarnoff; and her children, Josh Palmer and Eleanore Olszewski and Noah and Hana Palmer. Sara gives special thanks to her husband, Jeffrey B. Palmer, for his constant love, support, and patience; for his perspectives on parenting and disability; and for his insights on the art of writing.

# Raising Children—Resilient and Ready for Adulthood

------------------------------------------------------------

Kelsey and her husband are parents of an outgoing first grader who has spina bifida. The couple are best friends, confide in each other, and make joint decisions. By discussing their thoughts and ideas together, they help each other understand the advice of medical experts. They can support one another in pushing for more information when needed, and they can tap into each other's intuition when making decisions about their daughter's care. "At one point we felt that something wasn't right with her. We asked the doctor, and we were correct—our daughter needed surgery."

When Roberto's son Cory was 14, he was injured in a skateboarding accident and became paraplegic. Roberto was sad and upset—but not devastated—when this happened. Because Roberto's older sister has severe rheumatoid arthritis and lives a full life with a disability, he knew that Cory would still be able to reach many of his life goals—and embrace some new ones. When he returned to school after rehabilitation, Cory, formerly a soccer star, found a new role on the team—becoming the coach's assistant and co-strategizer.

Liz's daughter Janet was born with a disability. It broadened her view of the world. "It made me more knowledgeable. I had already crossed cultural barriers, coming from Scotland to Africa to the Midwest, with sabbaticals in far-flung corners of the earth." A divorced mother of two, Liz found that her daughter's disability required some special planning but did not prevent the family from traveling. Disability was just another part of their life equation. Janet, now an adult with a family of her own, shares her mother's passion for travel and adventure.

Kelsey, Roberto, and Liz raised their children—both able-bodied and those who have disabilities—to participate fully in life, not watch from the sidelines. They found ways to keep their kids healthy and safe—and to still include them in family activities, sports, travel, and other exciting life experiences. They prepared their children to handle life's challenges successfully and to become capable, independent adults. In short, they created *inclusive* families, building *resilience* in themselves and their children. And you can, too.

First of all, what is an inclusive family? It is a family that embraces every one of its members, including the child who happens to have a physical disability. Each person in the family is valued and respected as an individual and as part of the whole. His unique interests, talents, and aspirations are recognized and supported. Parents divide their attention fairly among all the children, and each child is loved, nurtured, and given what she needs to flourish. There may be times when the pressing needs of one family member are given more weight in the short run, but over the long run, the needs of everyone will be met. For instance, when Bobbi needs surgery to correct scoliosis or Elliot breaks his arm in a soccer game, their needs must get priority. But even in the midst of a crisis with one child, inclusive parents let each child know that they are loved and cared about. And after the crisis is resolved, an inclusive family returns to "normal" mode where every child's needs are given equal consideration. An inclusive family cultivates the sense of "I can do it!" in each child and strengthens their "rebound-ability," or resilience.

What, then, is a resilient family? Resilient families land on their feet no matter what challenges come their way. They go beyond merely surviving tough times: they adapt, rebound from stress, grow, and thrive. Parents in resilient families can meet their children's everyday needs, respond to unexpected setbacks, and anticipate challenges not yet on the horizon.

As psychologists with expertise in physical disability, we are particularly interested in the rebound-ability of families that include a child who has a physical disability. What are the keys to resiliency in these families?

Over the years, in our therapy practices and at national and local conferences, parents of kids who have physical disabilities have shared their stories with us. Their stories revealed their struggles and their successes and helped us begin to answer this question. To write this book, we also interviewed numerous parents, grandparents, and children in families that include a child who has a physical disability. Some families were more, and some less, resilient. Some had an easier and some a harder time including their child who has a physical disability in family life (and in life beyond the family). But each of these individuals inspired us with their love for their families, their tenacity in finding answers and resources, their openness to taking uncharted paths, and their generosity of spirit as they helped other families following in their wakes. And each of them taught us something about building resiliency.

Through a combination of these extensive family interviews, our own personal and professional experiences with disability, and concepts of resiliency outlined by other psychologists, we developed our own theoretical model for *creating an inclusive and resilient family when your child has a physical disability*. This model forms the backbone of the book.

Whether you are just starting out and "clueless" or a seasoned parent looking for a few new tips, this book aims to educate, support, and inspire you. The book explains the basic principles of inclusion and resilience, and it demonstrates the wide variety of styles and techniques that parents use to turn these principles into everyday practice. We hope this book also helps you become more resilient as a parent (and as a person), increases your confidence, and redefines what is "normal" for you and your children.

## How Parents Create Resilient Families

The hallmarks of resilient families are *pragmatism* (being realistic, down-to-earth, practical), *belief* in your child, and *vision* (seeing long-term potentials and possibilities). This combination of characteristics builds a sense of security, self-confidence, and a taste for adventure in children. Parents anchor their children in reality by *solving practical problems* in the here and now. They encourage their children to develop their talents, abilities, and self-confidence, by *communicating positive expectations* and belief in their children's strengths. They prepare their children for the future by *sharing their vision* of their children as independent adults and giving them opportunities to learn the behaviors and skills they will need to take on adult roles.

> Resilient Families   =   Pragmatism + Belief in Your Child
> + Vision of Child's Potential

$$\boxed{\text{Resilient Children} \quad = \quad \begin{array}{l} \text{Experience + Responsibility} \\ \text{+ Socialization + Risk Taking} \end{array}}$$

But sometimes, especially if one of your children has a physical disability, you can get so caught up in day-to-day practical problems or routines that you don't pay attention to what your children need to become capable adults. Many parents are highly capable in raising their children from infancy to early adolescence, only to have difficulty launching them into young adulthood because they haven't done the "prep work." Parents may find it scary to think about their children growing up, leaving home, and handling their own lives—and this is often true to a greater degree for their children who have physical disabilities. So, our model for raising resilient children emphasizes those aspects of life that parents need to structure for or with their children *throughout their childhoods*, in order to prepare them for life beyond the family when they become adults.

In our framework, there are four essential factors that prepare a child for life as a competent, independent, resilient adult:

1. participating in a variety of *experiences* that educate them about life;
2. assuming *responsibility* to build abilities and self-esteem;
3. having opportunities for *socialization* to help them form relationships with people outside the family; and
4. taking *risks* appropriate to their age to learn how to judge what is safe and what is not.

Competence in these four fundamentals is built on the foundation of an inclusive family—and developed in the context of each family's values and culture.

### Experience

We learn about life by being a part of it, by *experiencing* it. Do you remember taking your toddler out to walk in the snow, to feel the cold and hear the crunch under her boots, or visiting the beach, where your child sifted the sand through her fingers and put a toe into the surf? Remember that first fall when the training wheels were removed from the bike? These memories or experiences become your child's "book of knowledge" about life. When snow or sand or falls from bicycles are mentioned, your child knows the feelings, sights, smells, and other sensations. This knowing becomes a link to other human beings and the experience of life.

Providing this shared experiential language is a vital part of raising a child. There are countless realms of experience to which you can expose your child, from physical to intellectual to social, from artistic to philosophical.

Creating music and artwork, for instance, can be an important experiential part of a child's life. It helps a child make a design or object that didn't exist before; not only does the child create something unique, but in the process he figures out how to solve a variety of problems and shares his experience with others.

When you have a child who has a physical disability, there are challenges in providing equal exposure to life experiences for that child and your able-bodied children. Parents work this out in a variety of ways. The O'Briens, for example, encourage involvement in all types of sports and give music lessons to all of their daughters, knowing how vitally these contribute to each girl's self-concept. Sean O'Brien coaches his younger daughters' ball games and spends equal time horseback riding with his oldest daughter, who has a disability. In another family, daughter Jamie likes modern dancing, so she takes lessons, while her sister Brittany, who uses a wheelchair, takes adaptive dancing classes for both able-bodied students and those who have physical disabilities. Myron, a teenager who uses an accessibility scooter, takes classes at the local culinary school, while his brother Les plays soccer. Each family chooses either the same or different activities so that their children can experience the worlds that call to them. Families who strive to be inclusive, with or without children who have physical disabilities, generally follow the "rule" that when a door is opened to one child, another (though not necessarily identical) door is opened for the other children.

Many parents also help their children who have disabilities to have physical and sensory experiences of the world that might be difficult for them to do on their own. One father, in order to allow his daughter, who uses double leg braces, to experience what it felt like to run, put her feet on his and then ran with her. Running felt so exhilarating for the little girl that she cried when her father was so tired that he had to stop. Years later the daughter saw a young woman running across campus, her hair blowing behind her, and thought, "I know what that feels like."

In his fictionalized autobiography, Christopher Nolan, an Irish writer who had cerebral palsy, wrote poetically about the physical and emotional impact of experiencing a cold stream for the first time while on a family vacation:

> Certain chores had to be done and then the family moved over to the mountain stream. They washed and splashed but as ever Joseph [Nolan] was there too. Nora [his mother] lifting him from his chair handed him to Matthew [his father]. Barefooted he was let splash, let feel the wild, surging, frantic flowing water, let stand on the hard, cold, rock floor, and curl his toes and see how white and graceful looked his feet under the spring-cool water.

Nolan's parents realized his need to be in the world and experience it as others did, feeling the pulsing stream and the hard rocks on the stream bed; they made these types of experiences, and many others, available to him.

Some parents feel that it is equally important to give able-bodied siblings some experience of the medical or rehabilitation world that is an integral part of the life of their child who has a disability. Their children's encounter with what their sibling does in physical therapy, medical treatments, or recovery from surgery is educational; it answers questions and demystifies what happens. Experience is a two-way street.

Technological wonders open up new worlds of possibilities for your able-bodied children and those who have physical disabilities to participate together in many experiences. The sports world is a great example. For Lance Bowers, competitive biking is made possible by a hand-powered bicycle. Sit-skis tethered to experienced able-bodied skiers allow people who have disabilities to enjoy the world of snow sports. Others enjoy adaptive horseback riding. And as the Fisher family discovered, many water sports enjoyed by able-bodied kids can also be adapted for those who have physical disabilities. Swimming, boating, kayaking, and canoeing are some of the possibilities. Add scuba diving to that list: at a national meeting teenagers with spina bifida (SB is the most common neural tube defect) were taught scuba basics and tried them out in the water. Talk about I-can-do-it faces rising from the depth of the pool!

Advances in accessible sports open doors to inclusive *family* activities, but perhaps more importantly, they open doors for children who have physical disabilities to participate with their *peers*, building bridges through this shared experience. Wheelchairs and braces fade into the background when a 10-year-old who happens to use a wheelchair sit-skis with the class jock.

## Responsibility

All kids long to know they are valued and needed. They understand that others see them as reliable when they take on responsibilities that are appropriate to their age and ability levels. In years gone by children contributed to the family's survival and welfare by tending gardens or livestock, cooking, cleaning the home, caring for younger children, or making clothing. These chores gave children a sense of worth and were essential in building the skills they would need to assume adult roles in their own families. But at times this work was so strenuous and demanding that it left little time for them to play and be children. Even today, some parents assign so many chores to their offspring that their childhoods are stolen from them.

But in most of today's middle-class families, children's chores are much lighter—like loading the dishwasher or folding laundry. Yet the assignment of responsibilities is often a bone of contention between spouses, or between parents and children. In the families we interviewed, for example, some parents thought their children ought to be helping out more around the house, while their spouses felt that schoolwork, sports, other outside activities, and having some "down" time were more important than chores. In some families, academic achievement and participation in extracurricular activities take the place of home chores, becoming responsibilities for which children are held accountable. But in the long run, doing some work for the family's good builds each child's ability to be concerned and accountable to others. Think of all the things your kids could do using just a little of their time, such as setting/clearing the table, filling/emptying the dishwasher, sorting and running a load of laundry, cleaning the kitchen or bathroom, making a bed, putting dirty clothes in the hamper, feeding the cat, and so forth.

The prospect of deciding *how much* responsibility to give children at different ages, stages, and levels of abilities can create a quandary. You probably remember your mothers and fathers giving you a reasonable amount of responsibility to help with the family. Cindy, for instance, felt that her parents judged the amount well. She helped babysit her nieces and nephews, with gradual lessening of supervision. Eventually she took on jobs without oversight. She felt that this progression and the positive feedback about her babysitting prepared her for parenthood. Rose's mother encouraged her to build skills and self-confidence by teaching Rose to cook and make important decisions for herself, allowing her to take increasing responsibility as Rose seemed physically and mentally ready to accept it.

Some families easily find chores for their able-bodied children but are puzzled about how their child who has a disability can contribute. If you and your child are unable to find a way for him to do any of the chores mentioned above, what about having him keep the family calendar on the computer, answer the phone, read to or help a younger sibling with homework, or dig dandelions out of the family's lawn? You may assign chores, have the children volunteer for jobs from a list of options, or have them assign their own tasks. Jobs children volunteer for may surprise you because they may realize they can do more than you think they can.

Responsibility for self-care—grooming, choosing clothing, dressing, and gathering things needed for school—is taught early in many families. Your child may have added chores like bracing, physical exercises, or tak-

---

⚠️ Sometimes children who have physical disabilities are inappropriately given the job of "family therapist," expected to act as the go-to person for siblings, or even parents, who have emotional problems. In a group of teenagers, a young girl who used a wheelchair said that when her parents were going through a tough time, her family assigned her the job of "keeping everyone happy"—and she was feeling like a failure. This is not an appropriate assignment for any child—or adult; no one can be responsible for the emotional life of another person.

---

ing medicines. One mother taught her son to catheterize himself at age 7 so that he would be able to go to sleepovers with his pals and take care of himself without her help.

Of course, whenever you assign home, school, self-care, or other duties to your children, you will need to follow up and make sure your children's responsibilities are duly carried out.

## Socialization

Being social creatures, we are constantly building bridges to others. Some of us are very skillful at making social connections, and some not. Children's actual experiences of giving to and receiving from others help them build the social skills to begin and develop relationships, where they may find the common ground that leads to friendship.

We each have different degrees of the need to relate. Some of us are born extroverts, wanting to be around many people most of the time, while others are introverts, preferring a smaller group of friends and more time to be alone. Each social type can learn to hone his social abilities in the other direction; finding a middle ground between extroversion and introversion will often result in a more fulfilling social life. Remember that introverted children tend to feel fatigued when they have to put forth extra energy socializing with a large group of people, while those who are extroverts find it energizing to be part of a large group of people.

Understanding your children's social orientation allows you to support them in meeting their needs for social interaction. For instance, you can help your shy child by modeling social interactions, such as having her watch you make an introduction, or by letting her know that you sometimes feel shy or anxious, too. Share with her the skills you've developed to overcome that awkwardness. Make up some opening lines for her to memorize so that she'll have a quick initial hello, a handy tool to use when necessary. Let her know that she may need more alone time to re-stoke her social energy than her extroverted brother needs; her brother should know that the opposite is true for him—and that each preference is perfectly normal.

Parents set the tone for their children as they step out of the family and onto the broader stage, from neighborhood, to playgroups, to school. Your expectation that you and your children will accept others and, conversely, that others will accept you and your children communicates your belief in your children and in the basic fairness of relationships. If you are anxious about how your child will be accepted into the larger community, your uncertainty can be easily "read" by your child.

To widen your children's social circles, you might take some time to think about what skills your child will need at the next step of his development. Socialization can be challenging for any child, whether she is outgoing and friendly or shy and retiring. Many children experience teasing, exclusion from groups or cliques, or rejection by their peers for any number of reasons. You can help your child by first listening and repeating back what she is telling you to make sure you are getting it right. Then express your appreciation for your child's feelings, validating them so that she knows you respect her. Assure her that, although it sometimes feels like it, she is not the only person to have faced this situation before. By relating how all relationships sometimes run into rocky terrain and by modeling appropriate assertiveness, you can help your child learn to speak up for herself. For instance, when Jenni was "boycotted" by her third-grade playmates, she sought out the new girl in the class to play with, making the new girl feel included. Jenni's mother wisely advised her to avoid making enemies with her old friends, telling her that they would respect her more if she didn't react in an angry or spiteful way. Her mother's careful guidance and support led to Jenni's eventual readmission into her old group of friends. At the same time, Jenni helped bring the new girl into the larger group. Jenni's mother negotiated this terrain wisely. By keeping your cool when your child is upset, you can teach her valuable lessons in navigating social interactions.

For a child who is "different," because of his ethnicity, being adopted, or having a physical disability, making friends and joining groups can have an added layer of difficulty: it's hard to get others to see him *as an individual*, not defined solely by his "difference." Since social evaluations by others begin at first sight, a child's clothing, hairstyle, accessories, or makeup "speak" first. It is helpful to most children to look like other kids in dress or hairstyle in order to be one of the gang. For children from other cultural backgrounds or who have physical disabilities it is even more important to have similarities in order to bridge the chasm between themselves and the mainstream. Your child can further narrow the gap with others by developing unique interests or a good sense of humor to draw attention to the ways he is like others, rather than different from them. Perhaps he is into teen adventure novels or the latest singing group; these shared interests can outweigh the disability in the eyes of his peers.

On the other hand, it can be empowering to help a child find a positive place for her disability or other difference within her overall self-concept and personal identity. Adoptive parents of a child from a foreign country or different ethnicity can support his exploration of his cultural identity, even though it is not the parents'. For example, American parents can teach their adopted Chinese children about China or send them to "Chinese school." Similarly, parents can encourage their child who has a physical disability to think about how she wants to make disability part of her individual identity. For many children it will be desirable to see the disability as an important part of themselves—but not as the whole picture. It takes thought and some practice for children to accomplish this, to be able to say, "I am a girl who happens to have a physical disability; I am not a disabled girl."

### Risk Taking

Each child's "first"—of whatever!—widens her horizons and informs her and the world of what she can do. But every "first time" has its risks, whether physical or psychological. In reality we take a risk every time we step out the front door, say hello to a stranger, or walk across an intersection. As your child moves toward more independence, he'll need to take more risks, something that is exciting and frightening at the same time.

You may feel a little nervous when the topic of risk taking by your children comes up. Yet risk taking is inherent in life. It helps define our limits, what we are able to do and what is beyond our physical or emotional capacities. It can also result in the achievement of something we thought ourselves incapable of doing.

Risk taking comes in many forms and levels. From that first wobbly step, when you wish you could build a wall of foam for your toddler to fall into—especially if he wears tiny leg braces—parents find themselves wanting to make each new step a safe one. Coming to the realization that each step makes the next easier and surer helps us lessen our protective stance bit by bit. That first scraped knee hurts you as much as your little one, but you learn to cleanse and bandage the wounds that follow with the knowledge that they *will* heal in time.

Do you remember the first time you saw your child in the limelight, perhaps as an elf in the kindergarten holiday program? Knowing he was a bit shy, did you want to coach him through the songs? And then you noticed he was enjoying the rhythm and melody and had quite forgotten there was an audience. Fast-forward to tying his tie for his high school prom; he was eager to be on his way—while you sat at home, worrying about the after-prom party.

Parents of children who have physical disabilities share concerns about the risks we've discussed. But you have additional questions about your child's physical and emotional safety. For many, the very idea of risk taking brings to mind hospitalizations, fractures, and long periods of recuperation, not to mention the pain of demeaning remarks others might make to their children when they take the plunge into new social situations.

Parents, by and large, tend to be more protective of their child who has a disability than the child's siblings are. Several years ago a father and son got into a discussion about the fact that the father, newly retired, was driving his 23-year-old daughter, who used a wheelchair, to work every day. His son encouraged the father to let his daughter take public transportation to work. "But what if it rains?" asked Dad. "Well, Dad, she'll get wet, just like I do." Dad was most concerned with making life easier for his daughter, while his son was distressed that his sister was not encouraged to take reasonable risks that would allow her to be more responsible for herself. Brother knew that his sister was capable of growth toward independence, while Dad wanted to shelter and protect his daughter. Parents are wise to listen to siblings' opinions about the abilities of their brother or sister who has a physical disability, as they are sometimes more accurate in their appraisal of what their sib is capable of doing, and they don't carry the guilt some parents do.

As physical risk taking poses the possibility of injury, it is a hot topic for most parents. Weighing what is to be gained against the potential for harm of any action is a daily task for all of us. Even a risk gone awry can turn into a good thing, becoming a way to "normalize." For instance, at summer camp, Herbie, in his double leg braces, was riding a horse when it suddenly shied, knocking Herbie off. Herbie was very proud when he returned to school with his arm in a cast; he now had something in common with the other guys in his class, several of whom had broken their arms doing sports activities.

Jalah, who has OI, had a busy mother who gave her lots of freedom to make decisions about what she could do. She wanted Jalah to feel "normal" so she allowed her to bike and roller-skate. Her physician told Jalah's mother to "let her be a kid," even if it meant having a few extra fractures. Jalah sees this freedom to try out the world as a valued gift from her mother. She has tried to hand down this freedom to her son, Jon, who also has OI.

Kelsey's parents also trusted her to make her own judgments about safety and risk. She gained confidence in herself as a result and learned to trust her instincts; this was a "gift" from her mother and father. Other parents note that the trust their parents placed in them as children was translated into trust in themselves when they became adults.

Physical disability is an add-on challenge for you and your child, making it more difficult to assign responsibilities for him and help him join social activities, take considered risks, and learn from common experiences. While everyone has to get around some obstacles in life, individuals who have physical disabilities face extra hurdles, such as stairs, lost time from school for operations or medical treatments, and negative attitudes of others that limit their participation in normal life activities. The rest of this book will show you how you can create resilience in all your children, including those who have a physical disability.

## How This Book Will Help

So you have defined your goal: build an inclusive and resilient family. How do you do that? We will give you a broad perspective on families—yours and other's. Stand back for a moment to look at your challenge: preparing your children to become competent adults. Now that you have the foundation for the task ahead, the chapters that follow will take you from the moment you learn that one of your children has a physical disability, to coping day by day, and on to planning for your and your children's future. The perspectives and wisdom of real parents, grandparents, and siblings who may or may not have physical disabilities are included throughout the book.

Part I, "In the Beginning," explores how you learn about and cope with the new reality that your child has a physical disability. The focus of chapter 1, "Getting the News," is on hearing the words, at birth or later, that your child has "a problem," and dealing with the initial impact of a diagnosis of disability. It describes the spectrum of emotions—helplessness, sadness, anger, loneliness, and delayed bonding—that parents may experience and that grandparents and others close to them may also feel. Your first reactions to your child's disability and expectations for him or your family are explored. Out of this period of emotional tumult, parents discover strategies and inner resources that are helpful as they begin to take charge.

In chapter 2, "Coming Home," we look at adjusting to changes in the family routine when you have a child who has a physical disability, including changes in time and energy demands. In addition, emotional and attitude adjustments have to be made, and you'll need to learn how to deal with medical procedures and to communicate with rehabilitation professionals. During this process, you find that you are becoming an expert on your child's medical and disability-related issues and can become a partner with the professionals. As the process moves on, you will discover your family's "new normal."

Part II, "All in the Family," looks at the different perspectives of parents, siblings, and grandparents. Chapter 3, "Inclusive Parenting: Make It Work for You," emphasizes how you can reap the rewards of parenthood through creating your own unique family. The need for parents to build strong supportive relationships with their spouses or significant others, with extended family, and with the community is discussed. We explore how coping with your emotions and caring for yourself allow you to move on to the nitty-gritty issues of parenting, from time management skills to the expression of positive expectations for your child's success.

In chapter 4, "Brothers and Sisters: Siblings Sharing Family Life with Physical Disability in the Mix," the contributions and complexities of growing up with siblings, both able-bodied and those who have disabilities, are explored. By talking things through, sharing experiences, arguing, and helping each other, brothers and sisters build their "cope-abilities." Younger and older adults have found that their relationships with their siblings who may or may not have disabilities, in which so much was shared as they grew up, have a major influence on their values and beliefs, how they communicate, and how they support one another as adults.

Chapter 5, "Grandparents: Seeing through a New Lens," shows how grandparents can play a supportive role to their children and grandchildren when physical disability enters the picture. Depending on a grandparent's geographical proximity to his family and the extent of his resources, he can offer everything from emotional to physical to financial help. Grandparents can enrich the lives of their children and grandchildren, by being there for them and sharing their interests and talents. Many grandparents adapt to their new roles with renewed sense of purpose in life. Families point out that it is helpful to everyone if there are some boundaries between generations and a balance between emotional involvement and each generation's need to lead their individual lives.

In Part III, "Into the Wide World," the focus is on preparing your children for adulthood and yourself for life after parenting. In chapter 6, "Opening Doors to Inclusion," we discuss how to launch your children on the road to independence by giving them access to educational, vocational, and social opportunities and teaching them to manage their medical and physical needs, request accommodations in school and the workplace, and deal with the social barriers of stereotypes and negative attitudes. We explore the ways parents can balance dreams and reality to help their kids make plans for success in their future vocational and family lives, as well as how they can educate their kids who have physical disabilities about love, sexuality, and relationships, to prepare them for dating, intimacy, and marriage.

You'll see in chapter 7, "Letting One Dream Go to Let Another Grow," that as your children mature and begin to leave home, you'll find yourself moving on from on-the-job parent to empty nester. It begins with taking stock, gaining confidence, and trusting your instincts. By this stage you are balancing "I can do it!" with "Thanks for the hand!" and finding increased patience and tolerance in yourself. You may reconnect with your spouse or perhaps date again, plan a change of careers, return to work or enter retirement, spread your wings socially, investigate new hobbies or interests, or pursue a passion.

Interwoven between chapters are the stories of families striving to be inclusive. They represent a wide scope of family types with varying supports and challenges. Yet each is invested in the future of their children and has a strong belief in each child and in each parent. They share their unique experiences and perspectives on managing a family with both able-bodied children and children who have disabilities. They demonstrate the many ways that families can survive, cope, adapt, and thrive, while preparing their children for success in adulthood.

# PART I

# In the Beginning

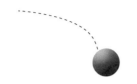

**The Webers:** A young family juggles the needs of twin boys, one with and one without a physical disability

Casey, a nurse, and Paul, manager of a large company, are the parents of Andrew and David, twin boys who will soon enter their tweens. Casey's pregnancy was normal, and each of the boys weighed over six pounds at birth. But while Andrew's birth was easy, David was breech. During delivery, his spinal cord was critically injured. In spinal shock, blue, and not breathing, David was intubated, whisked past Casey, and rushed to the neonatal intensive care unit (NICU). Casey recalls, "I thought I was prepared for parenthood, because of my mom. She was the great role model I was going to follow. But clearly I was not prepared to have a child who has a disability."

Casey waited six hours for the medical team to tell her what was happening. Initially they said that David was "not moving like a baby should"; several hours and several tests later, with Paul and Casey's mother, Elizabeth, in the room, the neurosurgeon told them that David had a cervical spinal cord injury (SCI).

As a nurse Casey knew exactly what this meant: "I immediately pictured my son five to ten years out as a quadriplegic. I almost knew more than I wanted to know. There is some truth to 'ignorance is bliss.' Having a medical background does help you ask the right questions. But being the 'professional' is much different than being personally involved with the disability. Your objectivity, to some degree, goes out the window."

When Paul and Elizabeth heard the news, they had little idea what an SCI would mean for David's life. Paul saw the fearful look on Casey's face and knew it was serious; he could hardly believe what was happening. His first impulse was to "hit the doctor," but Casey calmed him down; he "went home and cried." When Elizabeth grasped the seriousness of David's condition, she was also devastated; "as a grandparent, it's your child, too," she said.

Casey was shocked, sad, and overwhelmed. "I never once worried that something would go wrong. I was young and healthy and had a great pregnancy. Though I did know one of my twins was transverse in utero, all my doctors assured me it would be fine. When I found out he would be disabled for the rest of his life, I was devastated to say the least. For the first four days I was in the NICU with him I cried; I could barely speak to him over my tears because I was so distraught."

As the first grandchildren on both sides of the family, the twins were much anticipated. When Paul had to call his parents with the news about David, "it was hard to do. I made sure my Dad was home so I could tell my folks together." Paul couldn't answer many of their questions. His father flew out to be with them immediately, as did Casey's sister. The occasion of the twins' birth went from joyous to somber.

Grandmother Elizabeth had never been in a children's ward and found it wrenching to see David with a tracheostomy (breathing) tube. She often procrastinated, once not getting to the hospital until 11 p.m. But her son-in-law urged her to visit, and she understood how important her presence was to him and Casey.

David remained in the NICU for two months. Paul visited him at least once a day. He was still angry and filled with "ill will" toward the doctor who delivered his son and who he believed should have prevented David's injury. "I should have two healthy boys. It was depressing to see what the kids and their families were going through in the NICU. It was gut-wrenching."

Meanwhile, baby Andrew was thriving at home. Casey would "breast-feed him at home, pump extra for his next feeding, go to the hospital, feed and spend time with David, pump, and return home and do it all over again." She and Paul traded places so that while one was home the other was at the hospital.

Elizabeth had recently left her job with the understanding that she would return on an ad hoc basis in a few months. But when she learned about David's disability, she wanted to be available to help her family. Elizabeth's husband, on the other hand, believed that David would get better. "Why get upset about it?" he asked. She was frustrated by his denial of the serious issues David faced.

At first Elizabeth was unsure about her role. "I wanted to step in and do lots. Yet I didn't want to be interfering." While wanting to be respectful of Casey and Paul's role as parents, she soon jumped in to ask how she could help. She cooked, washed, fed the dog, dealt with everyday problems, and kept up normal routines, like decorating the Christmas tree while David was still in the hospital. She lived with Paul and Casey during this time, because her home was too far to commute.

When David left the NICU, he was sent by air ambulance to a rehabilitation hospital specializing in infants with SCI. After two weeks of intensive rehabilitation, he finally joined Andrew at home, where Elizabeth continued to help out. As a novice grandmother, it was "intimidating to care for someone with such elemental needs." But she soon learned how to provide David's daily care and familiarized herself with the full gamut of issues, from his medical and physical problems to the complexities of health care delivery and insurance. Elizabeth also became the second set of eyes and ears at medical appointments.

Paul lost his job two months after the twins' births, adding to the stress on the family. Casey recalls, "By the end of the year, we had no income and were having to pay for COBRA health insurance. I was forced to go back to work part-time." Their schedule centered on doctors' appointments, clinic visits, and daily home visits from therapists, nurses, and nutritionists. Looking back, Casey says she was on autopilot for the first two and a half years of her sons' lives. She thinks Elizabeth's help was their saving grace. "Her moral support, mom-education support (i.e., how do I do this?), and her help watching Andrew allowed my husband and me to be at the hospital together and to talk with the doctors." Paul agrees that extended family support is invaluable. "I would recommend that you live near your family. They are invested in you and your family and will help." Having a good relationship with each other was also important in helping Casey and Paul cope. "Luckily for us, my husband and I were fairly good at communication before all this happened. We were also dedicated to our family and knew we would do whatever it took to make David better. We continue to do that." Paul adds that many marriages can't survive "for better or worse" and says that couples have to work together. "You can't walk away and put the burden on a single parent." He likens parenting to a tag team, with success based on positive beliefs and creativity. Along with spouse and extended family support, Paul finds it essential to become involved in your community.

When the twins were 2½ years old, the Webers moved to another state where Paul found a new job, and as David stabilized, they settled into a routine. Paul's job gave them a steady income and good health insurance, so Casey could stay at home with the boys. This is when Casey "started falling apart" and Paul felt helpless. "There was nothing I could do to rectify this for her. I felt torn apart. I didn't know what to do or how to fix things. How could I get her over her depression?" Casey tried counseling and stress reduction classes. "They helped a little, but anti-depressant and anxiety meds helped the most by taking the edge off. I was then better able to organize myself, think, and relax."

Elizabeth, who'd "run on adrenaline" during David's early medical crises, had a period of emotional upheaval, when the boys were 6. "I had flashbacks to when the doctors walked in. It seemed to me they crawled along the walls and would have run away if they could. They did not want to deliver the news about David."

David's physical disability makes it challenging for the Webers to enjoy community and social activities. Playmates' homes have stairs and limited wheelchair accessibility. Playing fields and nature walks are often not wheelchair-friendly. Also, they need to prepare and bring supplies for David and time his bowel program to fit into their schedule. Everything has to be carefully thought out in advance; even the weather plays a role in their plans. During the summer, they can't go to amusement parks because the heat may cause David to have dysreflexia (a dangerous rise in blood pressure triggered by pain, temperature changes, or infection in people with SCI). For all hot-weather activities, they need to make sure there will be fans or air conditioning and cover from the sun. Some activities, such as scout hikes, are not possible for David; Paul says that when he thinks about what David is missing, "I want to sit and cry."

Nevertheless, Paul believes that life is to be lived, and the Webers—including David—participate actively in life as much as possible. "When you get past the 'woe is me' phase," says Paul, "you'll find that life has not stopped."

The Webers are major league baseball fans, like to go to movies, and take vacations. Both boys have flown with them several times to visit Paul's family. Because David's power wheelchair can be damaged during in-flight storage, they now take his manual chair when they fly—though this does limit his independence while they are visiting his grandparents.

Casey is the primary caregiver for the twins, but Paul is also involved with both boys and never hesitates to help with David's care. Casey's medical background is an asset in her role as hands-on care provider and "case manager" for David. She sets up appointments, orders equipment, gets supplies, and talks to insurance companies. "It's like a full-time job."

Casey and the boys have traveled to Washington, D.C., to increase awareness about paralysis and lobby their congressman to support related health care bills. When the twins were five, Elizabeth accompanied them on a trip. While Casey was at a meeting, Elizabeth took them sightseeing. At the Lincoln Memorial she sat on a bench while the boys chased pigeons. When they needed a taxi, the boys signaled the taxi like the doorman at the hotel did. "The boys have the expectation that the wheelchair will not deter them."

Elizabeth has lived through stressful times with the twins and feels closer to them because of it. She has gotten to know them well and finds them "delightful and normal. I love them to death." She takes them many places, making sure things can work for both of them. When the family was invited to a wedding reception, she checked the site out ahead of time and gave the manager a list of things needed to make it accessible for David. They were all done. "If no one had spoken up, nothing would have changed." Elizabeth also educates extended family and friends to make them aware of accessibility issues.

Elizabeth likes her children to tell her what they need. If she is overly involved, she wants them to let her know. She tries not to cross the line between help and interference. She encourages other grandparents, if they can, to put their lives on hold for a while in order to support their children and grandchildren in times of need.

The twins are close with each other. If he gets something for himself, Andrew automatically does the same for David. They do the normal things boys do; David likes to wrestle, using his upper body strength, and tries to trip his brother. Games and pretend play are important to them. They play Little League baseball, and Paul is one of their coaches. David pitches and has good coordination but poor strength; he gets to base in his wheelchair. He plays on two teams—one with his brother and one that is a special-needs team. Both boys belong to a Cub Scout den where Paul helps out.

Although not involved with organized religion before she had the twins, Casey wonders if it would provide good support for her family, especially David. Paul, though, has his doubts. He had a hard time "forgiving the Lord" after David's birth.

Casey feels that she is "definitely a different person today than I was prior to having a child who has a disability. The main portions of my personality remain; however, some things have changed for the better and some for the worse. One doctor told me several weeks after David was born, 'You can't let this change who you are.' I feel you can't help but have this change who you are. For the better, I feel I am more sympathetic or empathetic to others than I used to be. I do not take things for granted as I once did. I have used our experience with disability to be proactive and get involved in advocacy. For the worse, I am not as happy-go-lucky as I used to be. I worry. I get anxious. I get overwhelmed. I get angry. I get frustrated and exhausted from the excess care and attention David's disability entails. I feel at times like our life revolves around his needs. I have also realized I am more selfish than I thought I was."

Paul has high standards of behavior for both boys. His own upbringing shaped him to be a strict, no-nonsense dad. He doesn't like whining. He feels that kids in general "get off too easily" and insists that each of the boys has "to pull their weight." Paul and Casey are very clear, however, that Andrew is not responsible for taking care of David.

Casey feels strongly that as a parent you must meet every child's needs, but she finds that trying to keep things as equal as possible for the boys is a challenge. "The issue is how to balance the extra needs of an individual who has a disability with one who doesn't need as much assistance. They say the focus should not be on the individual who has the disability, but due to health and physical needs, it almost can't be helped. We try to incorporate it into our routine as much as we can." She wanted to spend one-on-one time with each child, "taking each twin on outings by himself." But she found that "the one-on-one time with the child who has a disability is to medical appointments, not fun activities. For the able-bodied child, the special time usually involves doing something fun. Plus, because they are the same age with the same interests, what I did with one was always something the other wanted to do. It always seemed unfair to leave one out. So my compromise is to always make time for something fun for the whole family to do together that focuses on our family as a whole unit." They do this by making play situations accessible so the boys have the same opportunities. If they can't adapt a situation, they don't do it. "We try to focus on what we can, not what we can't do."

But Casey also tries to take time each day just to sit with each twin, individually, and talk directly with him. "I was told early on, which I found useful, that it is not the amount of time you spend with each child, but the amount of quality time. It's not about going and doing, it's about paying attention to each of them and showing them both that I care about them, I love them, I respect them, I will always be there for them; they mean the world to me."

# 1

# Getting the News

--------------------------------------------------------------------

"We knew our baby had a hemorrhage, but I didn't expect the severity
of what was to follow."

—SEAN

"When my daughter got sick and suddenly couldn't walk, the doctor
was away and couldn't see her. She got weaker for two days, and then
we found out it was polio. I was devastated. I didn't know anything
about polio—and I was unhappy with myself that I was so remiss."

—CHARLOTTE

"Giving birth to a child who has a disability has pulled back a curtain
on a whole new world."

—LIZ

"Being a parent is a journey to the unknown."

—PILI

## Diagnosis: Hearing the Words

You can recall as if it were yesterday the moment you received the
news that your child had a physical disability. You may have been pregnant, or just given birth, or your toddler or teen had just had an illness or
accident. Hearing the words, noticing what was said or not said, feeling
the physical sensations, and being aware of who was there and who was
not are still clear in your memory even years after.

### Hearing the Words before Birth

Lola remembers hearing the doctor say that her first baby's physical
development was abnormal when she was seven months pregnant—and
the subsequent torrent of her emotions. Her husband Philip received the

news from Lola later that day. She was crying and upset, and he tried to reassure her. "I told her it would be the same, just different. I told her to go to her mother's; she was in shock."

Many parents recall their emotional turmoil when they heard the news that their babies would have spina bifida (SB), one of the disabilities more commonly diagnosed before birth through prenatal blood tests and ultrasound.

In the twenty-eighth week of her pregnancy, Priscilla Brandon hadn't felt her baby move and was sure something was wrong. Her obstetrician sent her for an ultrasound with state-of-the-art equipment. A number of hospital personnel congregated to observe the test, but no one said a word. Her husband Lee recalls that when they were later told that the baby might have SB, the doctor gave them the most "devastating worst-case scenarios. It was the worst day of my life." They were referred to a geneticist, whose news was equally bad. "Things are bleak," he said. "I have to prepare you; there may be brain damage." Priscilla cried for forty-five minutes after getting this news.

When she was five-and-a-half months pregnant, Kelsey learned through an ultrasound that her baby had SB. She remembers being offered the option of abortion and responding, "Absolutely not." At the same time, she felt that her "heart was broken. What did I do to cause or deserve this? Why me?"

Cindy discovered her baby's diagnosis of SB at her sixteen-week prenatal visit. While she knew people who were doing well with SB in her community, she says, "You never expect to have it happen to you." She had planned a celebration lunch with friends after the appointment but opted not to go. She chose not to tell people about the diagnosis; "I was still praying for a beautiful baby. I didn't want people to say, 'I'm so sad,' because I wanted this to be a happy time, and it was." Her husband had a harder time; after hearing the news, he was withdrawn and helpless, saying, "There is nothing I can do, I can't fix it." It was the only time Cindy had ever seen him cry.

Rose and her husband were thrilled when they became pregnant with their third child. They were shocked when they found out in Rose's fifth month of pregnancy that the child would have SB. Rose was depressed for a month. Her husband kept "his emotions close; he wouldn't talk about it. But he was stressed out."

When disability is discovered while the baby is still in utero, parents have some time to begin taking in the news, integrating the reality of disability into their physical and emotional preparations for becoming parents. They have time to learn about their child's disability, to develop some ideas of what life will be like, and to think about how they will include that child in their family life.

Priscilla and Lee, scared by the doctor's dire predictions for their baby's condition, decided to learn more about SB. Priscilla did research at their local college and found another specialist through the area's children's hospital. He explained to her that hydrocephalus associated with SB is treatable, and that brain damage can often be prevented. This information and the doctor's reassurance helped Priscilla and Lee develop a realistic, yet more optimistic, picture of what was to come. They began to experience some of the joyful anticipation that most parents feel.

Erica was six months pregnant when she and D. K. were told that their first child would be born with osteogenesis imperfecta (OI). They were both startled because the pregnancy had gone so well up to then. They went immediately into information-gathering mode, trying to learn as much as possible about OI and prepare for the birth. Erica admits that changing her expectations about her baby required some "psychological adjustment."

## Hearing the Words at Birth or Later in Childhood

Whether your child's disability was discovered at birth or later in childhood, you never forget the moment you heard the words, "There is a problem with your baby." Parents naturally feel vulnerable when threatened with the possible loss or disability of their child. Hopes can be unwittingly inflated—or destroyed—by the first words you hear from a nurse or doctor about your child's diagnosis and prognosis. Jim remembers how the doctor told him, "Your son may be a vegetable so you should find a good place to put him." "All I could think of was . . . an artichoke," he says, recalling the surreal experience. His son is now a strapping teenager who uses a wheelchair.

Diane recalls that her daughter was diagnosed with OI when she was 1 year old. There had been some signs at birth, such as darker sclera, but she appeared to be developing normally. It was only after her first baby tooth came in "opalescent" that a series of medical tests confirmed OI. X-rays showed evidence that she had had multiple fractures at some time during infancy (characteristic of OI), of which the family was unaware. "My reaction was initial sadness, feelings of loss, but there really wasn't time to dwell on it for I had a 2½-year-old at home to take care of. Learning my child had a lifetime disease that would hurt her and had hurt her was difficult to swallow. Not knowing she had both ulnas and a femur fractured—and in hindsight, remembering that I was present when it had happened—caused terrible guilt. However, being an optimist, I keep looking at the glass as half full. . . . I had two miscarriages before Rochelle and in some way I think that may have prepared me to be strong mentally and physically."

When your child is diagnosed with a disability, you may ride a roller coaster of emotions—sadness, guilt, confusion, anger, frustration. You may mistrust the doctor and perhaps deny the diagnosis, or blindly trust whatever you're told. You may feel incredible weariness, or be energized by a desire to escape or do something to make it better. It is mentally and physically fatiguing. You may say to yourself, "This can't be happening," "This can't be real," or "It will be different tomorrow."

For parents who have never known anyone who has a physical disability, or whose image of disability has been shaped primarily by negative stereotypes or media portrayals, adjusting to the idea of having a child who has a disability may be particularly challenging, whereas parents who are more familiar with physical disability through personal experience, such as having a close friend or family member who has a disability, may find it easier to cope with the diagnosis. They can more readily envision a life for their child in which disability is just one part, not the whole story.

Parents who adopt children who have physical disabilities have *chosen* to incorporate disability into their family life. They tend to have a more positive view of disability, although they may not be aware at the time of adoption of all the issues they will encounter as parents. Still, the initial impact for them is different. Like parents who receive the diagnosis during pregnancy, they are better prepared and do not have to do the re-imaging of their child. The child they have is the one they want.

Rachel and Donald could not afford the high cost of private adoption, so they became foster parents to children who had disabilities and then adopted them—six altogether! They were well aware of the challenges they would confront as the parents of children who had a variety of disabilities. They planned their lives around their family, and Donald took early retirement to help carry the load at home.

Frequently, only limited information about the physical condition or medical history of an adoptee is available to adoptive parents. Although they know that their child has some type of disability, they may experience some emotional upheavals later on if their child has unexpected difficulties with health or development or his disability diagnosis comes into sharper focus over time.

Of course, almost all parents, whether biological or adoptive, experience—simultaneous with their uncomfortable feelings—feelings of love for their children and the joy, pride, and exhilaration that go with becoming a parent.

### Ripple Effects of the News

When you throw a stone into a pond, you see concentric rings widening and spreading out around it. Like the ripples from that stone, the news about your child spreads from your immediate and extended family members, to your closest friends, to those not as close, and finally into your community. As parents, you feel the initial impact when the stone hits the pond. Your parents (your child's grandparents) feel the first ripple as they get the news from you and are filled with questions and concerns.

As soon as she knew her baby would be born with SB and hydrocephalus, Kathleen called her mother, Elsie, to tell her the news. Having no idea what the diagnosis meant or what to expect, Elsie was frightened. She wondered, would the baby live? How severe would it be?

Helen found out that her grandson would have SB when her daughter-in-law, Pili, was four months pregnant. "I was so sad. What's going to happen? A member of the family wanted Pili to have an abortion. I was so against that—but I was really scared for them."

Some grandparents absorb the impact more easily and are able to be supportive to their children right away.

When Joleen called her father to tell him his granddaughter had an as-yet-undiagnosed disability, he reassured her—and himself at the same time—that every child has "something." This baby girl might have a new kind of challenge, but they would find a way to handle it.

The next ring of ripples hits friends and then acquaintances as they get the news that your child has been diagnosed with a physical disability. Because friends are farther from the emotional center, they are often able to provide support, express concern and kindness, and help with reassuring visits, gifts of food, or perhaps babysitting for your other children. While Jada's son was in acute care following an automobile accident, her friend did research on the best rehabilitation centers for him to transfer to. She also told Jada about another family she knew who had gone through a similar situation and were willing to give Jada support.

But sometimes friends and family make assumptions about your feelings and needs—for instance, that you *must* be depressed, angry, or devastated—which may or may not be on the mark. This adds a layer of stress to the process of coping with the fact that disability is now part of your life. While you may not be devastated, you are probably using much of your energy to cope with your own feelings, to learn about your child's care needs, and to master the "medicalese" spoken in the hospital.

While it would be nice to have the wherewithal to respond to your friends' misconceptions about how you are actually affected by your child's disability, or to deal with *their* emotional distress, it is more important to reserve your energy for your child and your own needs. Later on, you will have the time and fortitude to answer your friends' questions, calm their anxiety, and correct their assumptions—if you choose.

# Responding to the Reality
## Initial Emotional Reactions

Parents of children who have physical disabilities experience a spectrum of emotional reactions, ranging from anguish to great happiness. They think about the disability in different ways, too—some see disaster, while others see opportunity. And many parents experience a yo-yoing of these feelings and thoughts, up one moment and down the next.

### Helplessness

Many parents experience feelings of helplessness or inadequacy after their child is diagnosed with a disability. Paul recalls "going home to cry" when his son was diagnosed with quadriplegia soon after birth. Paul's grief was mixed with helplessness and frustration; he could neither control what was happening to his baby nor comfort his wife in her own grief. "There was nothing I could do to rectify this for her. I felt torn apart. I didn't know what to do or how to fix things."

Andrea, whose son's rare disorder required multiple surgeries during the first weeks of life, had a similar experience: "I felt completely helpless. My baby was in pain and my husband was so sad, and I couldn't do anything about it."

Debbie, another new mother, didn't know anything about her child's disability. She felt inadequate and blamed herself, because she "missed the signs" and because there was nothing she could do to make it better.

### Loneliness

Parents frequently experience loneliness while coping with the initial diagnosis of a child's disability and the intense demands on their time and energy. One parent describes it "like a dark tunnel with little light and you just try to pick your steps carefully and take the right turns to get to the light at the other end. It is frightening." You may feel separate and alone. You may not have a confidante to whom you can turn for support, or you may be hesitant to "burden" your mate with your own feelings of vulnerability or fear. Sometimes old friends are awkward or unresponsive, not knowing how to be supportive. It feels like they desert you in your time of crisis.

*Anger*

Some parents experience anger in reaction to their child's diagnosis of disability. You may feel anger toward the medical staff, your spouse, God, or yourself.

When Charlotte was told the diagnosis of her 7-year-old, she was completely at sea because she didn't know anything about the condition. She felt "stupid" and became angry with herself because she knew so little.

Kathleen "couldn't wrap my brain around what was happening so I couldn't talk to anyone." Her doctor offered to get her help, but she was "so stubborn I wouldn't accept it."

Anger can become a "time bomb" for parents who have no opportunity to air their complex feelings about their child's disability. Sometimes parents are dealing with multiple stressors at the time their child is diagnosed—perhaps a divorce or loss of a job. The care of a child with many extra needs can leave a parent with no time to work through grief or loss. But parents can benefit from channeling their anger constructively. Runner, whose son Lance has a spinal cord injury, says, "My aggressiveness got me answers to questions." Anger motivated him to find the resources to help his son.

Harriette recalls some "gloomy days filled with anger" as she tried to cope with her son's multiple disabilities. But "when I saw that my anger was eating me up alive, I knew I had to direct my feelings in a more positive way." Harriette mobilized her "anger energy" to "nail down the benefits I had to have for my son's medical care and to get help at home."

## Separation from Your Child

Most couples expecting a child know that the *mother* may need medical intervention during delivery, such as anesthesia, episiotomy, or C-section. But most parents are unprepared for the possibility that their much-anticipated "bonding" time will be disrupted by the *newborn's* need for medical procedures or surgery.

Separation from their baby due to medical treatments right after birth is hard on new parents. The fact that your baby has been born with a disability may be less distressing than the loss of opportunities to feed, cuddle, and tend to your newborn. You may feel displaced as a parent by the health care providers who hold your child's life in their hands.

Kathleen had an ultrasound just hours before her baby's birth, which indicated fluid around the brain. A neurologist was consulted and diagnosed SB; an hour later, Kathleen gave birth. She got only a "quick glimpse" before they took the baby off to a specialty hospital. She felt as if she were in shock. "My baby was taken away immediately. I couldn't touch him or pick him up." In the specialty hospital, her baby was surrounded by medical machinery, nurses, and doctors, and there were strict rules about how to handle her newborn. "I felt like the nurses and doctors told me what I could and couldn't do. There were oodles of people around. Why couldn't I be alone with my own baby?"

Liz, whose daughter was also whisked away to another hospital for medical care, remained behind in the maternity ward, watching as the other mothers cared for their newborns. In order to get through the ordeal, she turned off her feelings, becoming numb: "I don't think I reacted very much."

When you are separated from your baby (or from your child, who is having surgery or a prolonged hospital stay), it's important to make extra efforts to reconnect emotionally. For Liz the first step was to recognize the feelings of loss she'd experienced when her baby was whisked away. Thankfully, their period of separation was short and they were soon reunited. Grateful to be with her baby, Liz held her close, fed her, and looked lovingly into her baby's eyes; she was emotionally open to her baby's needs and interacted with her as much as she could with a brand new infant. In this way, Liz set the tone of their relationship for years to come.

If you have to be separated from an older child, it is equally important to recognize *the child's* feelings (perhaps separation anxiety, fear of surgery or doctors, or loneliness) and to reassure him or her with a healing dose of TLC.

### Grandparents' Emotional Reactions

Grandparents are an important part of their children's and grandchildren's lives and can be a valuable source of support in good times and bad. While they want to be supportive, especially in times of stress, they may not know just what you need. They also have their own individual emotional reactions and may need some time to deal with them, so that they can be supportive of you and your family.

Elsie wanted as much information as possible after learning that her daughter and son-in-law's baby would have a disability; she asked her son to find out what was available on the Internet. At the same time, there was a sense of disbelief: "This can't be happening to us." Elsie asked herself, "What went wrong?" She also wanted assurance that her daughter and son-in-law would be okay. She worried about the impact of her grandchild's physical disability on her daughter's marriage.

Upon her grandson's birth, Elsie was thankful he didn't have brain damage. During the early days while he was in the hospital, she felt fearful about his future. What would he have to face? Would he be able to walk? Would he be accepted? "We were angry at first. But it also made us closer as a family." Elsie and her daughter were able to openly air their feelings, many of which they shared in common, and to support each other.

## Ways of Coping

Disability can rock your emotional boat up or down; what is tragedy for one family is triumph for another. We can view events, people, or experiences in our lives, including a disability, as *loads* or *lifts*. One of the tricks to coping with any difficult or novel situation is making the choice to focus on the lifts and to find enough lifts, or positives, to outweigh, or at least balance, your loads. Most parents find their lifts through trial and error, by testing behaviors, parenting styles, and coping mechanisms until they find the ones that work for them and their families.

It's common to focus more on the loads when you first learn about your child's disability. But even at this early stage, there are things you can do to change your point of view and look for the lifts, which will help you begin to move on from your feelings of loss.

### Sharing with Your Spouse, Partner, or Closest Friend

After the birth of your baby or when disability occurs in your older child, you seek solace, understanding, and an ear from your mate to "take

> Although it is difficult to summon the energy, reach out to the person closest to you—your spouse, partner, or family member. You may find that while you were trying to shield them from your feelings, they were doing the same for you. Acknowledging that you and your loved one are both experiencing emotional upheavals—whether in sync or not—can create a safety zone for each of you to share your feelings and fears.

in" and talk about your feelings and the "flipping over" of your expectations. (If you are a single parent, you can seek the same support from your best friend or closest family member.) But while you both need to reach out for comfort and support, you and your partner may have little time or emotional resources to give to each other. It may require all of your individual resources just to "keep your heads above water" and deal with pressing decisions about your child's physical needs.

You and your spouse or significant other may also be on different wavelengths, experiencing dissimilar initial reactions to the news about your child's condition. You may be out of "sync" emotionally, one feeling anger about the situation, while the other is denying the reality of what is going on. While this is common and expectable, it is important to keep your lines of communication open. Share your feelings with your partner and accept where she is on the emotional roller coaster. During these early stages mothers generally express feelings of grief or sadness and need time to vent and mourn; fathers more often express feelings of anger and want to take steps to change the situation. You both wish you could "do" something to control what's happening and to comfort each other, and it feels terribly frustrating when, at first, there seems no way to do either!

## Journaling

Even when you are still reeling from hearing the diagnosis, keeping a journal is helpful. If you don't have much time or feel too fatigued to do it in depth, at least make some quick notes that you can reconstruct later. Journaling about your feelings helps you unburden that weighty load of reactions you are carrying on your shoulders. It's also good to look back

> **T** If possible, keep all the medical information about your child, copies of doctors' reports, and information about medications, reactions, and surgeries in one section of your journal. Use another section of the journal as your "release" valve, allowing you to vent your thoughts and feelings about what is going on.

on later, to see how your feelings have evolved and gain some perspective on your experiences. This is especially helpful if you don't have a partner to share with.

You will be receiving lots of information about your child's diagnosis, how to take care of her physical needs (medicines, equipment, or procedures), and how to use the medical support system. The amount of information can be so large that you can't possibly remember all of it. Making notes in your journal can help you listen better and organize your questions when receiving new medical information and can jog your memory when you need to refer to the information again.

### Taking Constructive Action

Many parents cope with painful emotions by taking action—such as surfing the Internet for information on their child's condition, scouting out accessible facilities for family activities (curb cuts, ramps into schools, churches, theaters, restaurants), filling out insurance forms, building a ramp for a child who uses a wheelchair, or doing some other task that will solve a practical problem for their child or family. When Rose learned, while still pregnant, that her baby had SB, she dove into research on the condition and made sure she was fully informed about the latest treatments before her baby was born. She made arrangements to save her baby's umbilical cord stem cells, in case they could be used in the future to promote better function. Over the years, Rose has kept up with all the latest research and treatment innovations, and her daughter will soon be participating in a clinical trial of experimental nerve rerouting surgery.

When D. K.'s son was diagnosed with OI, he did not allow himself a "pity party." He, too, turned his sadness into action, immediately searching for treatments and cures and gathering information about the practical side of dealing with the disorder.

Taking action shifts your attention toward a more positive attitude and results in greater productivity and feelings of accomplishment. Moving from a stance of helplessness to active problem solving helps parents regain a sense of control over their lives and emotions, at a time when everything seems upside down. As one dad said, "The more choices and control you have, the more easily you'll accept and cope with the situation."

## Getting Social Support

Take advantage of emotional and social support offered by friends, extended family members, coworkers, or professionals, especially early on when you've just received word on your child's situation. This support helps you feel less alone in the world and strengthens your resolve and ability to take effective action when it is needed.

Gary spent many weeks at the hospital after his newborn daughter had surgery to correct a hole in her heart. His friends were busy working, and most wanted to avoid the distressing experience of visiting the pediatric intensive care unit (ICU). But Gary developed close relationships with other parents of kids in the hospital and soon had a small network of supportive peers. These connections gave him a chance to unburden himself and, later, to get advice about accommodations for his daughter at school and how to find home health aides for her.

Early on, Cindy talked with her friends and also reached out on the Internet to people with similar issues. The voices of experienced parents about how they coped with the initial diagnosis and birth gave her some good ideas and made her feel more supported. These relationships continue to help Cindy maintain her equilibrium and perspective on life.

Rose recalls that right after her baby was born, the hospital staff was "awesome, because they were so professional." The staff suggested that she attend support groups in the hospital even before she took her daughter home. These were helpful to her in coping with her initial emotional reactions to her daughter's diagnosis. They also gave Rose contacts for mental health counselors in case she needed additional help.

## Spirituality

When hearing difficult news, most people are sustained by the faith or belief system that has helped them in the past. There is comfort in the known and trusted, and for some parents, this includes spiritual or religious beliefs.

The first question formed by many parents, "Why me, God?" may be both a prayer and a demand for understanding. Some parents find relief, perspective, a sense of hope, and support through their spiritual beliefs or practices. These benefits can come through meditation, prayers, "talking with God," or simply a belief in a benign higher power.

Cindy, whose religion is a source of strength for her, "felt compelled to talk with a priest; he listened and we prayed." Her parents also prayed for their new grandchild, and their priest talked about him at Mass. "I asked for strength to be able to handle this," Cindy says; "I didn't ask for it not to be."

Nasim, upon receiving the call that his son had been paralyzed in an automobile accident, was devastated. He contacted his mosque immediately, and by the time he reached the hospital's ICU, his imam was waiting at the hospital with his wife and her parents. He consoled the family and led them in prayers. Nasim felt that Allah must have some plan for his son. His faith helped him find hope and convey to his 14-year-old son a sense of meaning and purpose.

After hearing during pregnancy that her child would have a disability, Lola contemplated having an abortion. But she heard an inner voice say, "Trust in life." This spiritual experience, which she accepted without question, helped prepare her to accept and love her baby boy born a few months later.

Not all parents believe in a higher power, and parents can certainly find strength and confidence without spiritual beliefs. Alan, for example, did not believe that God had any role in the fact that his son was born with congenital deformities. He simply had "no use for God." Alan felt that it was up to him to carry this load alone—and he firmly believed that his lack of reliance on a higher power made it easier for him to tackle problems and make good decisions.

When her daughter was diagnosed with juvenile rheumatoid arthritis, Rebecca rejected the visits of the clergy to the hospital room. "I have my own beliefs about life and its origins, and they do not include spirituality. I rely on my own inner resources. I know that I have ultimate responsibility for my life; when the doctor gave me the final diagnosis, I knew I would deal with it. I didn't need a higher power to depend on."

After getting the news about their child's disability, parents experience a wide range of emotional reactions, but soon they begin to find ways to cope with their feelings and the practical aspects of this unexpected situation. Around the time that your child comes home from the hospital or rehabilitation center, another phase of family life begins. As you integrate your child's disability into the everyday life of your family, you can anticipate making some changes in your family's activities, attitudes, and timetables. You may need to learn how to provide hands-on care for your child and to manage ongoing physical or medical problems, and you will develop new ways of thinking about your children and your family. In time, all these changes will become routine for your family, as together you find your "new normal."

### *The Hamiltons:* Raising teenagers in a blended family with humor, responsibility, and respect for differences

Evelyn and Scott Hamilton have three children, two from her first marriage and one from his. Evelyn's son Mark is a college student. Her daughter Celeste and Scott's son Richard are both in high school. Scott and Evelyn first met in high school. They dated, broke up, and dated again in college until Scott changed schools. They kept in touch sporadically and were reunited years later.

While still in college, Evelyn met Romi, a foreign exchange student. She became pregnant and married him soon after. Both continued their studies. Romi had a modest student stipend and played in a band at night. Evelyn's family would not help her financially after the marriage, so she had to work. She felt alienated from the rest of the world, pregnant "out of wedlock" and married to a foreigner. Romi slept late during the day and refused to help when their son Mark was born. Evelyn took comfort in her relationship with Mark and found joy in exploring the world with him.

When Mark was 4, Evelyn gave birth—alone—to a daughter, Celeste. Romi was playing a gig that night, as he had been when Mark was born. A physical exam immediately after birth revealed that Celeste's left arm had broken during delivery, and further tests showed multiple fractures in various stages of healing. The sclera of her eyes was blue instead of white. Four hours later, Evelyn was told that Celeste probably had osteogenesis imperfecta (OI). Celeste was flown by helicopter to a specialty hospital.

Evelyn and Romi followed by car the next day. The diagnosis of OI was confirmed. Romi felt responsible, in part because the family doctor incorrectly told him that OI was more common in children of Romi's ethnicity. Romi never held Celeste; their closest encounter was when he moved her from one spot to another. Even when he was alone with Celeste, he avoided touching her.

Evelyn felt abandoned by her husband and her family, who maintained their distance even after Celeste's birth. Friends, too, stood back, hesitant to help care for Celeste because they feared harming her.

Evelyn wrote to her old friend Scott about Celeste's birth. "I panicked," Scott recalls. "I didn't know how to respond. 'I'm sorry' was insufficient. I didn't write back." A year passed before he sent an apology. Evelyn responded, and they began to communicate regularly.

Meanwhile, Evelyn was entering a whole new world of medicine and rehabilitation. Her experiences with Celeste's medical care were "almost all good," but there were some rough times. Many doctors did not accept Medicaid, the only insurance the family had. As a result, Evelyn had to do her daughter's splinting herself. Finally, they were directed to a Shriners Hospital where they found a doctor with expertise in OI, a helpful social worker, and financial assistance to buy equipment for Celeste. Because of these positive experiences, Celeste has little fear of medicine, needles, or hospitals.

Because Romi had become so remote and uninvolved, Evelyn managed life for the children on her own. "I had to grow up really fast. I was doing all the research about OI as well as being the primary caregiver. I was the one in charge, assertive, determined, focused." The upside of this was becoming a better parent, says Evelyn. "It improved the way I parented my son, too." She filled their free time with art, concerts, parades, balloon festivals, and movies. But there was no adult "time-out" because she could not find day care for Celeste.

Evelyn was very conscious of Mark's needs, too. She "didn't want him to become an adjunct of his sister. I had an older sister, second of five, who was given the job of caretaker. She didn't get a real childhood. There was too much stress put on her by our mother." Evelyn made sure that Mark did not become "a slave to Celeste's disability."

One day she discovered an online support group for OI. The other mothers were empathic and offered practical advice on caring for Celeste. Two weeks after joining the group, she started taking Celeste, then a toddler, off the pad where she spent all her time. She found that Celeste began to move around more.

Around this time, Romi's behavior went from remote to threatening, and Evelyn feared for her children's and her own safety. She took the children, moved to her father's home in another city, and soon filed for divorce.

Meanwhile, her friend Scott was on the down slope of his marriage. Although he tried his best, it ended in divorce. A year later, he and Evelyn got together. When Celeste was 5, they married. Their marriage has been close and supportive. Scott loves to make Evelyn laugh, and he "keeps me stable so I can take care of the kids."

Scott now joined the new world of disability and medicine. He and Evelyn followed the advice they'd been given by an easygoing doctor to "let your daughter lead you." They asked Celeste to tell them how to do things so they wouldn't damage her. For instance, Scott asked Celeste, "How can I pick you up?"

Blending the two families was rocky at first. Scott's son Richard stayed with them some weekends during the school year and for an extended time in the summer. At first, Richard and Celeste did not interact. He saw her disability as foreign and a hindrance to having fun. Early on there was a three-way wrestling match, and Mark and Richard clunked heads with their sister. Their parents abruptly put an end to this physical play. Richard said Celeste "spoils all the fun." But as the years have passed, Richard has acclimated to his sister's disability and the siblings have become friends.

Evelyn and Scott are open about their differences in parenting, particularly on the issue of risk taking. Evelyn's son Mark is allowed to take risks within reason; he's able-bodied, thoughtful, and able to judge the risks and benefits of most situations. Scott says that not too much is off-limits with either of the boys. Richard and Mark participate in a variety of sports and physical activities. But Scott is more cautious with Celeste: he is aware of the time a broken bone requires to heal and is afraid of letting Celeste do things that could cause a fracture.

Evelyn wants Celeste to take some reasonable risks, like going sledding and bike riding, where the chance of injury is not too high. When Celeste was small, Evelyn would throw her up in the air and catch her in the pool, just as she did her son. She says Scott can be a "dream crusher. He seems to say 'I love you so much I don't want anything to happen to you.'" Scott has relaxed a bit since Celeste had an operation to put rods in her thigh bones, resulting in fewer breaks. He and Evelyn have taken

Celeste ice-skating in her wheelchair, with Scott pushing hard to make her go fast.

Celeste likes the thought of being close to the edge and feeling the wind in her hair, but at 15 years of age, she hesitates to take risks posing bodily harm. Now Scott's main concern is about her driving a car. "I worry about who gets to her after a crash. Paramedics might harm her, won't know how to take her blood pressure, for instance." Scott is also worried about Celeste's medical care when she goes to college. He fears she will need extra help if she has a break. He wants to have an emergency backup plan, and he hopes she will attend a school close to home so her family can step in if necessary.

Evelyn is more concerned about Celeste having a good social life and wants her to drive for that reason. Celeste is very sociable, a good writer, a violinist, and a Girl Scout. As a child she had more friends, but as a teen, her peers often "blow her off" or cancel plans at the last minute. Evelyn and Scott want Celeste to fit in like everyone else, but also to stand up for her rights. Celeste once told a boy off in the cafeteria for making rude remarks about her. Other students stepped in to stick up for her.

Scott and Evelyn have also encountered some people's negative responses to Celeste. Scott says there are times when he wonders if anyone notices or cares. But then they go into a shop and someone won't stop staring at their daughter. While Evelyn is offended because "Celeste is not on display," Scott sees these situations as "an opportunity to educate." Evelyn disagrees. "I didn't sign up to be a spokesperson for OI. I just want to get my stuff and get out."

As preparation toward independence, all the kids have responsibilities around the house. Chores are matched in time and effort, with Mark and Richard doing the heavy lifting and moving, and Celeste helping with chores such as using the Dustbuster. "We believe in fairness in the world, and no one receives special privileges," says Scott. Evelyn agrees that letting Celeste get off easy, or doing everything for her, would not be helpful. The more she does, the more strength and stamina Celeste will have.

The Hamiltons express affection and cope with stress through laughter and kidding around. "Humor is the primary language in our home," says Evelyn. Sometimes, as a lark, when they are all in the car they will group text chat on their cell phones. Scott's favorite times are family dinners or Sunday brunch, when within minutes everyone is goofing off and joking—a veritable "laugh riot." Scott knows that there is a delicate balance between individual and family needs, and he encourages each child to do solo activities. But in the final analysis, Scott's focus is on family togetherness.

Evelyn believes she still has much to learn about being a parent, but she tries to treat her children as individuals, to recognize their different personalities and help each one become what they want to be. She's also learned the importance of "taking care of myself so that I can be a better, whole, capable person. Parents need to be well rested to do a good job and make good decisions. That makes a big difference in the kids' lives." Evelyn has been pleasantly surprised by how much she enjoys being a mother. "Parenthood defines me," she says; "I love it."

# 2

# Coming Home

-------------------------------------------------------------------

"I quit work. I didn't have as much freedom as other young mothers because my baby needed catheterizing."

—KATHLEEN, MOTHER OF SON
WITH SPINA BIFIDA

"There was an adjustment period. His older sister was jealous because he got 'extras.'"

—MARY, MOTHER OF SON WITH
CEREBRAL PALSY

"I put one foot in front of the other. I did what needed to be done. I closed out feelings and concentrated on the next thing to do."

—ABE, FATHER OF A DAUGHTER
WITH CEREBRAL PALSY

"I got more chores but I didn't mind doing them."

—VINNY, OLDER BROTHER OF
A GIRL WITH CEREBRAL
PALSY

When your child finally comes home from the hospital, you feel relieved but nervous at the same time. What's in store now that responsibility for your child rests solely on your shoulders? Some misgivings and fears are common. Life can feel a little different than it was before—or totally "out of whack." You'll confront unanticipated problems that sometimes feel insurmountable. But little by little, you will learn how to manage.

You'll find that challenges come on two levels, the practical and the emotional. Practical problems can be solved with concrete actions, things you can do that have visible results. These might include learning how to care for your child's physical and medical needs, restructuring your work and family schedules, and adapting your home for the needs of your child who has a disability.

Emotional adjustments can be harder than changes in your physical environment or routines. While you physically "put things in their place" by making your home accessible, you'll find it more difficult to do the same with your emotions. Physical fatigue can accentuate feelings of sadness or frustration. You'll need to find some time for rest and a way to make "space" for your emotions, to recognize and cope with them constructively. Eventually, you'll learn how to "put disability in its place," not letting it take over your (or your child's) life.

This chapter explores a number of practical and emotional changes that families experience as a child's disability becomes part of their daily life—new time and energy demands, different family activities, accessibility issues, and getting help from others. It looks at how to manage your child's ongoing medical and self-care needs, work with his medical team, and become an expert on his disability. And it describes the experience, shared by many parents and siblings, of finding a "new normal" as they embrace a child who has a physical disability into their family.

## Adjusting to Changes in Family Life
### Time and Energy Demands

Parents in families that include a child who has a physical disability wish they had additional hours in their days to do everyday tasks—getting ready to go somewhere, going to the bathroom, dressing, eating. And they note the extra demands on their physical energy. For instance, Pili needs extra time to put on her son's braces and organize the special equipment she needs to have on hand for him whenever the family goes out. Their daily schedule must include time for Pili to catheterize her child every five hours and to locate safe and accessible places to do so. Liz, a single parent, recalls the time and energy demands of caring for her baby daughter with spina bifida (SB). In addition to parenting, Liz continued to work as a writer and college professor; she was tired all the time.

You and your partner and family will need to set priorities to avoid overloading yourselves. Making changes in your work hours, increasing the amount of help you get from others, or simply letting go of less important chores are all ways to cope with the increased demands on your time.

Kathleen gave up her job outside the home to care for her children, and she also missed out on many social events because of her baby's complicated bladder catheterization and bowel care regimens. Kathleen couldn't hire just any babysitter or nanny; caregivers had to be specially trained. Support from her mother and husband helped Kathleen make the transition to being a full-time mother. "I'm not mad," she says; "it's just the way it is."

Runner and April wondered how they could manage 4-year-old Lance's unpredictable and complicated treatment schedule without one parent at home full-time. They weighed various alternatives and decided that Runner would quit his job while April kept hers. Although their income was reduced, their stress was, too. They enjoyed a better quality of life, and Runner loves the extra time he has with his son.

### Getting Help outside the Family

Whether you are a single parent or have a partner, extended family and community members can help you lighten your load and make it easier for your family to cope after your child returns home from medical treatment or rehabilitation. They can support you emotionally, physically, and sometimes financially. All parents can benefit from help; some can receive it graciously, while others find it hard to accept.

Angie has "a million friends," says her mother, Mia. "So many people have helped with meals or money. When someone does something for us, it is hard for me to receive their help. I was always the helper; I was the one who cooked for others and gave them money. It's my family pattern."

You might find it upsetting, as Leigh did, if outsiders jump in to help your family without asking whether you want or need assistance. When Leigh's neighbors wanted to throw a fund-raiser for her daughter, Leigh felt angry, thinking the neighbors viewed her family as "needy" and unable to handle her daughter's situation. Even well-meaning neighbors can go overboard when they assume that a family whose child has a disability must be in dire straits. But most neighbors offer to help out of kindness, not because they think your family is incompetent. It is helpful to communicate your wishes to others and let them know when you feel you can handle things without their help. But it's also important to leave the door open to accepting—or asking for—help in the future, should the need arise.

Susie initially found it difficult to accept kindness from others. As a single mother with four little boys, two who had physical disabilities, she had to rely on help from her friends, but she felt uncomfortable with being beholden to them. But she learned to accept help when one of her friends told her, "Someday you'll help someone else, and in that way you'll repay me."

Bobby, whose son lost an arm in an accident, found it easy to accept the help that was offered by his friends and church members. "What goes around comes around," he says. "I've always volunteered with kids at church and helped my neighbors rake their leaves in the fall. So I figured it was my turn—and boy was I grateful."

## Family Activities

Many families that include a child who has a physical disability make some changes in the types of things they do together. Sometimes the child who has a disability needs more hands-on help with an activity than the family can provide, or has limitations in how much he can participate in leisure activities that his siblings or parents enjoy. More advanced planning is necessary, reducing spontaneity. Mia says, "It's tough. You can't just run off. We used to go camping but haven't since Angie was born [with osteogenesis imperfect (OI)]. We have to keep her safe." You may need to make adjustments in family outings and vacation plans so that all your children are able to enjoy sports, games, and recreation. Every family has different ways of doing this. You might want to focus on leisure activities that are accessible to *all* members of your family or can be adapted to include your child who has a physical disability. Finding a substitute activity that can give everyone the same excitement or exercise as their old favorite will make this work better—you might take skiing off your list, for example, and focus on water sports and sledding, if they are more accessible or adaptable for your child. Another approach is to give your children who are able to ski the chance to do so and find an equally attractive activity, perhaps horseback riding, for your child who has a disability.

## Accessibility

A step is not just a step. There is an old pamphlet with a picture of Itzhak Perlman, the famous violinist, standing with his crutches at the bottom of a flight of steps, saying, "I hate steps!" If you are a parent of a child who cannot climb steps, you understand the depth of meaning behind this statement. Steps, curbs, very steep inclines, and other architectural barriers can convey, particularly to a child, the message that he is unwanted or unworthy to enter. A mother of a son who has a disability says that she has only one friend who has a house without steps. Although she can carry her son up the stairs now, she knows that she will not always be able to do so. How will that limit his ability to hang out with friends at their homes as he becomes a teenager? One solution is to make your home the gathering spot for your child's friends. You might also invest in a portable ramp to use when visiting homes or other places where there are only a couple of steps. Friends might ask about how they can open up their homes; you can refer them to information on "visit-able homes." These homes are based on the barrier-free, universal design concept, meaning they can be used by both able-bodied people and those who have disabilities. Inclusivity is the goal.

## Adjusting to Changes in Yourself
### Dealing with Your Emotions and Attitudes

Parents need to deal first with the practical aspects of caring for their children after they have a baby who has a disability or an older child has a disabling illness or trauma. There is no time or energy to analyze your emotions when you are swamped by the physical and medical care of your child, especially if you have one or more other children at home. And

> ☛ Grief, loss, and other "negative" emotions are normal. These reactions don't mean that you love your child any less or that you are a "bad" parent. Allow yourself to experience these feelings before trying to "get over" them. Grant your spouse, family, and friends the permission to do the same.

> **T** *Working through feelings.* Releasing your feelings, whatever they are, by sharing them with a friend or a counselor can bring some relief. Remembering that feelings can change from moment to moment and that you don't necessarily need to act on them makes them less frightening. Facing your feelings and dealing with them will free up energy for you to better support your child. Crying, sharing your frustration or disbelief, getting mad, and telling your story—perhaps many times—will lighten your load and ease your discomfort and confusion. Allowing yourself to replay, refeel, or rethink your situation will make your feelings less intense, and with time they will gradually fade. As you gain distance, you will develop a new perspective.

you may not be *ready* to deal with emotions that threaten to overwhelm your ability to function in the heat of a crisis. But after your child is at home and life is humming along, your emotions may come back at you full force.

Casey felt sad when one of her twins was born with a spinal cord injury (SCI), but she quickly had to "get with the program" to care for them. A couple of years later, when her family life was finally in order, Casey "fell apart." Like Casey, when you finally have more time and energy, you may experience a delayed emotional reaction to the stress of your child's initial illness and hospitalization. Some people become more depressed, others more nervous or irritable. Some parents have delayed reactions and difficulty accepting their child's disability as a result of negative attitudes about disability or expectations that will not be fulfilled. Understanding and working through these difficult feelings takes work and requires support. It is necessary work, allowing you to gain strength and perspective in order to see and appreciate your *whole* child, who is so much more than his disability.

Although parents often have anxiety after coming home from the hospital, it may occur during other transitions, for instance, when their child who has a disability gets an infection, is assigned a new health aide, starts school, has an operation, reaches puberty, goes to camp, or leaves home for college. Paul, whose son David has complex care needs due to quadriplegia, says there are "so many things to worry about on a daily basis.

Sometimes I feel like I'll lose ten to fifteen years off my life span because of this stress!" Some parents of kids who have physical disabilities worry excessively about their children getting hurt, either physically or emotionally, as the children take steps toward independence. Terry, for example, whose 17-year-old son Jamie has severe juvenile rheumatoid arthritis, was surprised when her husband talked about finding a college with accessible housing for Jamie. Terry assumed that Jamie would live at home and go to a local community college and had even daydreamed about building an apartment on their house so Jamie could live there "forever." Scott, whose stepdaughter Celeste has OI, gets anxious about her doing anything that could cause her physical harm. His wife, Evelyn, describes him, at times, as a "dream crusher," holding back Celeste out of fear of her getting hurt. Anxiety overload can lead to overprotecting your child, preventing him from experiencing life to the fullest. Talking with your partner or co-parent can help you to reduce your anxiety and increase your tolerance for the risks your children *need* to take.

You or your partner may have negative attitudes or stereotypes about physical disabilities which you learned somewhere along the line. Maybe you were horrified when your child was born with or developed a disability but were able to put your attitudes on the back burner immediately after her birth or during his acute illness. You may find them surfacing again after your child comes home, you develop a set of daily routines with him, and the reality of disability sinks in. You may have prejudices against people who have disabilities, or perhaps you had negative experiences with disability in the past. If you see your child's disability as a reflection on yourself, you may feel angry at your child or view his disability as your personal failure. If these attitudes prevent you from bonding with your child, being a good parent, or enjoying the experience of parenting, you can use some help.

Sam had polio as a child; now a senior citizen, he recalls that his mother saw his disability as an embarrassment and a personal "blow." His father, less concerned with his physical abilities, expressed pride and excitement about Sam's academic achievements. This positive attention from his father helped Sam maintain his self-esteem and achieve success in school and his career, in spite of his mother's negative attitudes.

If you are unable to change negative attitudes that get in the way of nurturing your child who has a disability, even after getting support from a spouse or other adult, you should seek professional help (see below).

## Charting Your Emotional Progress and Getting Help When You Need It

One of the ways you can better understand your emotions and attitudes and chart your progress in coping is to keep a log or journal of your reflections and feelings. In your journal, you can pour out emotions and thoughts without someone judging you. Reviewing your journal periodically can show just how far you have come in improving your mood, your attitudes, or how you relate to your family. Or it might help you catch a downward trend and recognize when you are struggling and in need of help.

If you are running an "emotional fever" for more than a week in a row, it's time to look more closely at what's going on. Are you lacking

---

*Feelings thermometer chart.* On paper, rate yourself on a 10-point scale from 1 (none) to 10 (most intense) on your feelings of sadness, frustration, isolation, anger, being misunderstood, exhaustion, or other feelings you may have. Take your emotional "temperature" by rating yourself on the 1 to 10 point scale. Retake your "temperature" several days in a row. At the end of this time, look to see if there is an upward or downward trend or if it is stable in one spot.

☛ Sharing your feelings with someone you trust is a powerful way to release your feelings, to hear them and assess them. This person can be a friend or family member who is a good listener and can accept your feelings without judging you or dictating how you should deal with them.

momentum to get the laundry done or schedule a date with friends? Are you physically exhausted, depressed, or overwhelmed? Do you need more support from others?

Sometimes you need more than a friend to change your negative thoughts or help you find a way to move forward. Don't be afraid to seek professional help if you find yourself in this situation.

Choosing a therapist who is best suited to your needs is important. Try to get two or three recommendations and call each therapist for a short phone interview to determine your comfort talking to them and if they have experience working with people with your needs. To prepare for your first session, make a list of your feelings, concerns, and questions ahead of time so you don't forget to tell the therapist about them. You will probably feel relieved after the first session because you have taken the hardest step toward changing the way you are feeling.

Grandparents go through their own emotional adjustments as they come to terms with a grandchild's physical disability. Feelings of loss, anger, sadness, and anxiety, among others, are common and to be expected, just as they are with parents. Grandparents may use denial to protect themselves from the emotional impact of a grandchild's disability, or try to reverse events by bargaining with God. Parents' and grandparents' emotional reactions may not be in sync: mother is sad while dad is angry, grandmother thinks everything will get better, and grandfather is full of nervous energy and wants to get going on building ramps. It helps to remember that each individual's feelings are okay and that where a family member is emotionally at any given moment won't last forever. Emotions will change, and you will all move on in time. Rose's family is an example. When her child was born with OI, her husband's family was supportive, stepping in to help care for their two older children and soon to take all three children in order to give the parents some rest. They made their new little granddaughter with OI part of the larger family's life. Rose's mother,

> If you feel stuck, find professional help. You might choose to work with a psychologist, social worker, counselor, psychiatrist, or pastoral counselor. Advocacy organizations and state organizations for various mental health professions can recommend experienced therapists. Friends may also be able to recommend someone to talk with you. Remember: you are not "sick" if you ask for professional help; you are a good problem solver!

on the other hand, had a difficult time adjusting to the fact of her granddaughter's disability and did not help out. After a while, she did sort through her feelings and became a part of the family support team.

When Kelsey was five months pregnant, she told her father, Ned, that her baby had SB. Ned and his wife started reading about this condition and found only negatives. Ned was frightened. "I had a hard time dealing with it. My brother had muscular dystrophy. I didn't know if I could handle this again. I associated hospitals with death, but that changed with Leeann and her surgeries. She adjusts and we adjust. She has had twelve surgeries and is now a candidate to walk. We had to live with it to find the positives."

Despite differences in emotional reactions and timetables, grandparents can be incredibly helpful to your family when you are adjusting to life after the hospital. Many grandparents are willing to educate themselves about your family's emerging needs and help you build an understanding of the complex new situation you face.

Pepere and Memere, grandparents of a child with OI, had previous positive experiences with physical disability before their granddaughter was born. Although they "would have been happier or more relieved had she been born healthy," their past history had given them a good appreciation for the reality of living life with disability. The experience of Memere's brother's life with quadriplegia after a car accident "had already provided us a foundation of compassion and understanding." Their view that disability is just one factor in a person's life, that it doesn't dominate his existence, and that he can enjoy and experience life gave their granddaughter and her family strength and hope to cope with and move beyond their initial fears about OI and disability.

## Managing Ongoing Medical Problems

When your child comes home from the hospital, his medical condition is probably stable. But it is likely that he will continue to experience medical complications or surgeries, or need extensive treatments or rehabilitation therapies—for several weeks, months, or years. This is another new fact of life, one you will cope with better as you gain experience.

Parents who go through repeated medical crises with their children—bone breaks, respiratory problems, or surgeries—find that the first episode is often the most trying because everything seems foreign and overwhelming. Often there is no blueprint for what to expect, what to do, or how to respond. But after living through the experience, you learn that your child—and you—can do it!

While your own experience and growing confidence will make things easier, having a good relationship with your child's doctor is also essential to getting good care for your child and supporting you in caring for your child's medical needs. Look for a doctor who is empathic, reassuring, and positive. He or she should be a good listener who can understand your painful emotions and respond to your concerns about your child. Ideally, your child's doctor should include you as a partner in the medical care of your child and boost your confidence in parenting, while providing reassurance when you need it. Your doctor's support for your dream of creating a happy family is invaluable.

---

*Going around the cone.* Picture one of those orange cones used to direct the flow of traffic. The bottom is the widest part, and from there it narrows to a point, so that each time you circle it, higher and higher, the circumference grows smaller. Similarly, the first go-around with a child's medical crisis is the most difficult, as you have to learn a great deal of new information and at the same time deal with strong emotions. You'll find that when this medical issue comes up again, it will be less stressful because you're more prepared. You'll know which tools and strategies can bring you full circle, and you'll get to the end point sooner. The trip around the cone grows smaller with each circle, and each time around you can manage the situation better—both physically and emotionally.

---

Priscilla's baby was diagnosed with SB while she was pregnant. She couldn't imagine how she would cope until she found a doctor who told her, "Wait until you have this beautiful baby. You're going to love him and play with him and cherish every moment you have with him. Leave his medical care to me." This put everything in perspective.

## Communication with the Medical Team

Medical care for your child who has a physical disability usually involves more than one doctor. To be successful in navigating complex health care systems and becoming an active participant in your child's health care team, you will need to develop an effective way to communicate with multiple providers and hospitals or rehab centers.

Each parent has a different way of working with medical providers. One study described parents' styles of relating to the medical team along a continuum, from those who try to keep as much control over their child's treatment as possible ("confrontive questioners") to those who accept and go along with every medical recommendation without question ("compliant consumers"). Between these extremes are the "managing partners." These parents form a partnership with the medical team; the parents can make the final decisions about their child's care, but they have the benefit of frequent access to the expertise of the providers.

Any of these styles can be effective at different times and in various situations. When your child has an emergency, you may be more inclined to go along with the doctor's recommendations, but when you have time to consider and choose a treatment from several alternatives, you might want to ask more probing questions about the pros and cons of each choice. A "managing partnership" with your child's health care team is ideal in most situations, although at times you may want to give more weight to the medical team's advice, or at other times you may need to advocate for your child and clearly express your wishes or views, perhaps differing from those of the medical team.

As a parent, you need to know how to handle your child's daily medical care needs, and you probably learned much of this while your child was in the hospital. But now you will have to decide when to seek urgent medical attention and when you can manage on your own. And if your child has an illness, symptom flare-up, or surgical procedure, you need to know how to provide any extra care that's required. As a parent, you are responsible for monitoring changes in your child's condition and communicating with your child's doctor—and for asking questions, expressing your concerns, and voicing your opinions. When you communicate well with your child's doctor, you will develop a mutually trusting relationship and learn to put more trust in your own ability to provide your child's medical care at home and to make good medical choices for her when necessary.

By the time their son was a youngster, Priscilla and Lee were comfortable expressing their concerns and anxieties, asking questions and seeking information from his medical team. If something didn't sit well with them, they could speak up about it. Once effective communication had been established, they were able to rely on the medical team for a sense of security. For example, when they were worried about their son's new pressure sore, the nurse reassured them. "It's okay. It's not major; we'll keep an eye on it." This type of feedback helped them learn that they "didn't have to be alarmist."

Sometimes parents are shy or embarrassed about admitting their confusion, discussing their fears and concerns, or challenging a doctor when they disagree with his opinion. But if parents don't speak up about these things, there can be misunderstandings that lead to serious problems. For Evelyn Hamilton and her first husband, Romi, poor communication with their daughter's doctors led to years of needless guilt and worry.

When his daughter was born with OI, Romi was told that OI occurs more frequently in people of his ethnic group. This information was inaccurate, and it was presented to (or heard by) Romi in a way that made him feel blamed for "causing" his daughter's condition. He felt so guilty and so afraid of hurting his daughter that he rarely touched her. But Romi neither discussed his guilt or fears with his daughter's doctor nor sought other professional opinions or new information about OI. Sadly, this misunderstanding led to increasing physical and emotional distance between Romi and his daughter.

Evelyn, too, suffered for years from a misconception about her daughter's condition. Early on, she received a report of her daughter's genetic testing and misread the numbers coding her daughter's type of OI—she thought it was the most severe type, and for a long time she expected her daughter to die before reaching adolescence. But she never tried to confirm the genetic typing with her daughter's doctor. Years later, when she had to get her daughter's health records to travel overseas, Evelyn discovered her error—and she cried over her "wasted pain."

Things can be especially muddled when a child's disability develops over time and the cause is unclear. Multiple specialists are consulted in these "difficult cases," making it harder for parents to keep track of complex medical information. Communication gaps between the various doctors are also common. Ironically, getting an accurate diagnosis is sometimes *more* difficult when multiple specialists are consulted. This is what happened when Marie's daughter Ashley was injured.

Marie recalls, "I was at work when the call came; I dropped everything and was at the scene in twenty minutes. Ashley was standing there, talking to the police. The car was totaled. She had a headache and was in shock. I took her home." Though Ashley walked away from the accident, three days later she started experiencing bouts of paralysis, involuntary shaking of her body, headaches, and pain. Her parents took her to the ER and told them about Ashley's accident, but a CT scan did not show any injury. Over the next several months, Ashley's condition deteriorated, and she couldn't walk or get on and off the toilet by herself. She saw numerous specialists, but none could make a definitive diagnosis. Ashley thought she heard one doctor say that it was "all in her head," which was disturbing to her. In retrospect, she might have heard him say that she had a mild head injury and misinterpreted his meaning. Another doctor suspected she had transverse myelitis, a disease that damages nerves in the spinal cord. Ashley's inability to walk and do her own personal care led to a stay in an inpatient rehabilitation hospital, where a comprehensive evaluation of her physical, cognitive, and functional abilities led to the final diagnoses of lumbar SCI and postconcussive syndrome.

When the diagnosis is unclear, parents experience the pain of knowing that something is wrong, yet *not* knowing what it is or what the effects on their child or family will be. Sometimes there really are no concrete answers, and you must live with an uncertain diagnosis, do what you can to care for your child, and hope for the best. Unfortunately, when a specific diagnosis has not been made, parents (and kids) may get the message—intended or not—that their child is being "bad" or "acting crazy" or that they are not doing a good enough job as parents. This can damage your (or your child's) self-confidence and contribute to a delay in making an accurate diagnosis of a significant medical problem. In these situations, trust your instincts about your child. As a parent, you know your child best, and if you don't think he's a bad kid, then he probably isn't. Your confidence in him and in yourself as a parent will reassure your child and help you become her advocate. You may need to do some additional research to find a doctor or medical center that can find the reason for your child's symptoms.

Jane's son, Adam, was born with his umbilical cord wrapped around his neck and had to stay in the hospital for six days. He was susceptible to infections as an infant, and they were in and out of ERs for seventeen months. When he was 2 years old, Jane's car was rear-ended, and Adam was hurt. He had been potty trained before the accident but "regressed" afterward. Jane took him to a neurologist, but his diagnosis was unclear. When he was 6 and still unable to control his bladder, she took him to a urologist, who told her that Adam was just "lazy" and "not disciplined." But Jane firmly believed that she was a good mother and that Adam was a good kid, not "lazy." She continued to search for a diagnosis, taking Adam to a number of different specialists. Finally, when he was 8 years old, an MRI showed a cyst in Adam's spinal cord blocking the nerve signals needed for bladder control.

Adam's spinal cord condition is expected to worsen over time, with eventual paralysis of his legs a possible outcome. But now that Jane and her husband have a clear picture of Adam's diagnosis and his expected function, they can make better decisions about how to manage his current symptoms and plan appropriately for his future. Jane advises parents to get a second opinion and not to "take what is said in the hospital as gospel."

After understanding the cause of their child's disability, parents want specific information on the likelihood of the condition improving or worsening and on its long-term effects (prognosis). When information about prognosis is unavailable or confusing, many parents feel more unsettled

---

☞ Remember that no other person possesses the broad perspective and intimate knowledge of your child that you have. Trust yourself to do what's right for your family. Although you can benefit from the advice and input of professionals, ultimately, you must decide what's best for your child.

---

and anxious. The more detailed this information is, the better you can plan for your child's and family's future needs. Again, it's essential that you keep asking for this information and not give up or accept ignorance. You may have to ask for a separate appointment to speak with the doctor by phone or in her office, because she is probably pressed for time during regular clinic visits. Or you might need to take your child to a specialty hospital or clinic to get clearer information about his prognosis.

Casey had a medical background and knew that her son, who was born with an SCI, would most likely be permanently paralyzed. "I almost knew more than I wanted to know," she recalls. Still, like other parents who are less sophisticated about SCI, Casey needed to hear about her son's prognosis from "the horse's mouth." But she remembers "sitting in clinic waiting rooms for hours, waiting to see a host of doctors to get very little information, other than he is 'doing fine.' Most of the answers to my questions were, 'We'll just have to wait and see.' No one could tell us what his outcome would be."

After moving to a different city with a specialty hospital for kids with SCI, Casey finally felt that she was getting answers; even though she was hearing mostly what she already knew or suspected, it was validating to have confirmation from the experts, and it made her feel more understood and cared about.

### How to Get Answers to Your Questions

Most medical professionals who care for kids who have disabilities are well informed and compassionate. They will work diligently to find the best treatments for your child and be responsive to your questions and concerns. If you are frustrated with your child's medical care, consider whether there are ways you can improve the situation. For example, try restating your concerns and questions so your needs become crystal clear. When you have a suspicion that something is wrong with your child, bring it to the doctor's attention and insist on getting her input.

If you don't understand what a doctor is telling you, try asking him to repeat the information using different or simpler words, or to give you written information or instructions. Don't be hard on yourself if you don't "get it" the first time; most parents find that it takes some repetition to absorb complex medical information.

Lynn, who has three daughters who have disabilities, worked in a hospital. She came to parenting with a good medical background, yet she had to pose many types of questions to her children's doctors in order to extract the specific information necessary to manage their medical needs. "This is a good skill I learned in childhood," she says, "to find another way to ask the question." Lynn emphasizes the importance of getting the answers "in language people understand."

One way you can learn to ask better questions is by doing some of your own research at a library, on the Internet, or through the consumer organization for your child's condition (see the Resources section of this book). Once you've read and thought about the information, you will have a much better idea of what you are dealing with—and what you *don't* know. You can then organize your questions, write them down, and bring them to your next doctor's appointment. It helps if both parents make a list; often each parent will think of different but equally important questions. It's a good idea to list *all* your questions and concerns, no matter how trivial they may seem.

Scott, whose stepdaughter has OI, says, "I always do my homework. I go to the doctor with an idea of what's wrong and which options the doctor will present. It is important to me to always ask why he is making a recommendation. It seems you've got to know about the specifics of the disability because of the potential for a bad decision."

## Becoming an Expert on Your Child's Disability

One way that medical and rehabilitative care has changed over the past thirty years is that patients (even children) and their families are included in medical decision making more than ever before. In the course of parenting a child who has a physical disability or chronic illness, there are many decisions to be made regarding medical care, surgical procedures, and rehabilitation. Some of these will be no-brainers, like whether or not to set a broken bone. But others, such as whether your child should have a leg-lengthening surgery or a course of experimental therapy, are much more complicated. Such decisions require consideration of your child's and your family's goals and values, emotional and support resources, insurance coverage, and other factors. Understanding the medical information provided by your child's doctors is just one piece of the puzzle. You may need to learn more about your child's insurance and disability benefits, social and community support services, assistive technologies, and educational options, in order to make the best decisions and plans. Casey recalls playing simultaneous roles, as "a mom, a caregiver, and a case manager," while attending to her son's medical needs, negotiating changes in their insurance coverage, and trying to make ends meet on one income.

In addition, parents—and other family members—play a central role as "hands-on" care providers for their children who have disabilities. Fifty years ago, children who had severe physical disabilities living in urban areas were more likely to attend "special" schools or live in institutional settings, frequently with children having intellectual as well as physical disabilities. Now, due largely to advances in disability rights legislation, including the Americans with Disabilities Act (ADA), children who have disabilities are cared for in the "least restrictive environment," and there is widespread recognition that most children who have physical disabilities are healthier and more successful when integrated into regular public or private schools, just like their able-bodied peers.

The ADA requires public schools to make accommodations for kids who have physical disabilities, and participation in social and leisure activities is a major goal of medical rehabilitation programs. Other changes in the medical system, including limited insurance coverage for professional caregivers, shorter hospital stays for acute illnesses and rehabilitation, and the increasing specialization of medical care, contribute to the greater role that parents play in the home medical care of their children who have physical disabilities.

Parents of children with complex or unusual medical conditions often learn more details about the condition than are known by any one of the many medical specialists who care for their child. Parents frequently become the "case coordinators" and information specialists on their child's disability. Parents in these roles find it helpful to collect and store information on their child's medical history, surgeries, and current symptoms and make sure it gets distributed to all of his doctors. One father who has a son with complex medical needs keeps a spiral notebook in which he puts all doctor reports, medication and treatment changes, schedules, and problems that arise. You may also need to educate nonmedical service providers (such as teachers, counselors, and aides) and extended family members about his medical needs and care.

Diane and her husband learned as much as possible about managing their daughter's OI—mostly from the OI Foundation—and then they educated their extended families. "The doctor called us after seeing the X-rays and told us of his suspicions of OI, Type 1, and within minutes we had located the OI website, which explained so much. Finally, all of her issues made sense. The dots were connected; everything was clear. We read and read and read—and then we passed the information along to our families."

D. K.'s family, including a son with OI, has moved around and traveled a great deal. If his son needs care in an area where there are no OI specialists, D. K. sometimes instructs the doctor on how to treat him. To further his efforts at educating medical personnel naïve about OI, D. K. printed information about the diagnosis and laminated it to the back of business cards. He is now able to give these out to new doctors and others involved in treating his son.

At times, educating yourself, your family, and your doctors can be exhausting. Becoming an expert on your child's disability—and sharing your expertise with others—takes a huge amount of time and energy. Parents struggling to raise a family, including the extra care needs of a child who has a disability, have a heavy load to carry and shouldn't expect to be "perfect parents" at all times. If you are able to learn the basics necessary to care for your child, and if you are willing to ask questions when you need more information to handle new situations or decisions, you are doing a great job. If, like D. K., you can also bring fact sheets and treatment plans to your child's doctor, give yourself extra credit!

Grandparents may be able to help you gather information or come up with creative ideas about your child's treatment. Weighing the pros and cons of medical decisions is one of the hardest tasks for parents of

> ☞ Stress and anxiety are common when your child is having ongoing medical problems or requires extra care. Remember that there is a connection between your mind and body; stress (or "de-stressing") in one area affects the other. Next time you're worried, try smiling. You will find that your facial muscles relax and, more importantly, the "worry tape" in your head stops running. Pretty soon your body is more relaxed, too. Creating a new and positive mantra or repeated message for yourself is another way to control anxiety—for example, "Things are tough but I can do it." (Repeat as needed!)

kids who have disabilities. Your parents (your child's grandparents) can support you by sharing any information they have found in their own research; when a grandparent has done his homework on a particular treatment, he can make an important contribution to the discussion. Grandparents may also help simply by being the sounding board as you discuss the pros and cons of various treatments.

Sometimes a grandparent feels strongly about a different course of action than you are inclined to take; hashing out your conflicts can help, however, by forcing you to reexamine your decision and be sure it still feels right. Ned, grandfather of Leeann, notes, "I don't always agree with what's going on. I fought against Leeann getting a feeding tube—but it has helped her put on weight. She has reflux that I blame on the tube because she didn't have it before." Still, Ned knows that many factors have to be considered in judging whether the benefits of a treatment outweigh the side effects—and that, after stating his position, a grandparent needs to step back and accept decisions that parents make for their child.

## Partnering with Professionals

Marie's introduction to the medical system came when her daughter Ashley had a car accident at age 17. Ashley's medical situation was complex, but as Marie discovered, her insurance coverage was equally complicated and difficult to manage. Marie's biggest frustration during the initial months after Ashley's injury was the fight with her insurance company for coverage of Ashley's extensive medical care and rehabilitation. "I am angry at our medical system. We had been insured for years, with no claims. And then when we need that support, they won't put out. It's not right!"

Like Marie, many parents find it next to impossible to fight on two fronts at once—advocating for the best care for their child and arguing with insurance companies to get it covered. You may be more successful in your efforts to get various services and insurance benefits if you partner with a social worker or case manager. Help is available from several sources (aside from physicians) within the medical system itself, as well as from community-based support groups, consumer health associations, and social service agencies outside the medical system.

Within the medical system, social workers, counselors, psychologists, and psychiatrists are frequently available, either as a regular part of your child's medical team or as consultants whose services can be requested by the doctor. Social workers can help you with many of the practical aspects of making medical decisions and providing care for your child, including insurance coverage, financial assistance, hiring caregivers, finding rehabilitation, educational, or vocational services for your child, and so forth. In some settings, social workers also provide counseling to help you cope with emotional stress and complex decision making. Social workers (who are called "case managers" in some settings) also work for many county or state governments and are sometimes assigned to work with families in the community who are dealing with disability, medical crises, or financial hardship.

Rehabilitation counselors have special training and expertise on disability. They can help you or your child with emotional or social problems related to disability, help you communicate with social service agencies, and help you find the educational and vocational services your child may need. Rehabilitation counselors are on the staffs of state departments of vocational rehabilitation, some rehabilitation hospitals, community-based family service agencies, and college campus offices on disability.

In addition to these practical concerns, your child might benefit from professional mental health services to help him cope emotionally. Your doctor may suggest these services if your child is clearly in an emotional crisis or having extreme stress, but children are not routinely offered mental health services just because they have a physical disability.

Jon, a 33-year-old man with OI, is seeing a counselor for the first time and finally getting the benefit of psychotherapy. He recalls that as a child "kids teased me, treated me differently. I couldn't play sports. I had no coping mechanisms; I just felt bad. I'm a fairly screwed up adult because of it." Jon thinks he could have used some therapy when he was younger, but his family was overburdened with problems, including his parents' divorce, his father's alcoholism, and Jon's physical problems related to OI. They were too overwhelmed to deal with his emotional needs on top of all that. While Jon feels that he became stronger in some ways because of his disability and the need to care for himself emotionally, he also regrets that he "can't accept help from others, as I feel it is weakness." Now a married man, one of Jon's goals in therapy is to learn how "to open up, to accept help emotionally from my wife."

Many parents, with fewer social problems than Jon's family had, are so overwhelmed by a child's medical and physical care needs that, even when counseling is available, they are unable to take advantage of it. Psychotherapy can often be expensive and is not fully covered by insurance. You may be concerned about your child's mental health but not be able to afford the cost of psychotherapy for her. But don't give up—psychotherapy may be available at little or no cost at community mental health centers in your area, or through pro bono (that is, no cost) programs run by nonprofits or mental health professional associations.

Recognizing and communicating your child's emotional needs to his doctor or health care team is advantageous. Early counseling or therapy can sometimes prevent a crisis from developing, and many children who are not mentally ill can still benefit from counseling to help them cope with emotional and social stresses.

So if you think your child would benefit from counseling or psychotherapy, *ask for it*. Your child's doctor can refer you to a psychologist, social worker, or counselor, or you can locate a psychotherapist through hospital clinics, community clinics, or private practices in your neighborhood. Don't hesitate to tell a private psychotherapist if you're not sure you can afford his services; many practitioners have a sliding scale fee structure, adjusting their fees depending on the parent's income.

### Peer Support and Education

Many parents and families find education and support through peer groups. Some of these are for families of children who have specific ill-

☛ Other parents of children who have physical disabilities have walked this path before you and are a great source of information. If possible, find other parents of children your child's age with whom you can "co-trailblaze." Parents of children older than your own may also be able to help you by charting what lies ahead.

nesses or disabilities, and some include parents of kids who have a variety of different disabilities.

Pili, the mother of a child with SB, says that counseling from a professional would have been helpful "up front," when her baby was first diagnosed. But although counseling was not available, she found that valuable support "came from other families." She is active in a support group and says, "It's incredible to share your journey with parents of kids who have other disabilities, not just spina bifida. It is good to have someone you can connect with."

Peer support groups can help you become an expert on your child's disability. They can be found through many consumer health organizations, hospitals, rehabilitation programs, and social service agencies. Many are listed in the Resources section of this book.

## Finding Your New Normal

Once your family has made some adjustments to the routines of daily life and worked out a way to manage medical problems when they resurface, life begins to settle down a bit. Your focus shifts away from narrow medical and disability-related problems and broadens to include the interests, activities, and relationships that make up normal family life. Despite the media stereotypes of disability as a family tragedy or a badge of heroism, your child who has a disability is an ordinary child—and your family, a "regular" family.

Part of creating this new "normal" for your family involves limiting the role of disability in your child's life and in yours. As an inclusive parent, keeping your child's disability in perspective will allow it to gradually become part of your family's scenery, rather than taking center stage.

> ☛ Maintain a balance of friends who have children with disabilities and those with able-bodied children. This can lessen your feelings of "apartness" or "specialness." It is important to keep the perspective that all children have the same basic psychological and social needs and most parenting and growing-up issues are the same for both able-bodied kids and those who have physical disabilities.

When this starts to happen, it will be easier to focus on your child's needs *beyond* his disability, to give equal attention to all your children, and to take better care of yourself.

As parents, you are not alone in creating a sense of normality for your family. Your other children play a central role in this process. Especially when their brother's or sister's disability was present from birth or started early in life, siblings tend to view the disability as simply a fact of their family life, rather than something weird or a cause of emotional distress. Research shows that people who have one or more close relationships with a person who has a disability have more positive attitudes toward disability and are less likely to view disability as the defining characteristic of a person. This seems to apply to siblings, who often have positive attitudes toward their brother or sister who has a disability and see them as capable, reliable individuals. Most siblings define their inclusive families as "normal."

Erik, whose family includes three younger sisters who have physical disabilities, is right on target when he says that each family has to define its own "normal." Erik's mom and her partner chose to grow their family by adopting daughters who have disabilities, but the family makes room for Erik's needs as well. Disability is a big part of their lives, but not always the main act. Erik's family rejects outsiders' interpretations of their lives; they are comfortable with themselves as a family. "What is normal?" Erik asks. "My family is normal."

Jean thinks of her older brother who has SB as her "best friend" and says, "Disability is normal to us, part of our daily routine." Sukey, the youngest of five sibs, was born years after her eldest sister had polio. She experienced her older sister as "just normal. She was my wonderful big sister who happened to walk on crutches." Paige says that the only times she thinks of her sister as having a disability are when medical questions come up about her care. Otherwise, "she's just my sister."

Able-bodied siblings may look up to their sib who has a physical disability for her exceptional strengths in coping with disability, but more often they value the same personality traits, talents, or intellectual achievements that would make any sibling admirable. As the younger brother of Albert, who has an SCI, Terry thinks it will be difficult to duplicate the achievements of his sibling: "He's a great student, a leader, and is really popular at school. I don't think I will ever be able to do all that he has done." Fred remembers how he "rode on my younger sister's popularity." He dropped his sister off in her wheelchair at middle school each day as he drove to high school. She was well known and liked, and Fred, who was quiet and a bit shy, liked the recognition he received as her brother.

Siblings also understand that a brother or sister who has a physical disability is not mentally limited, and they respect their sibs' intelligence. Zoey recalls that when her baby sister was born with OI, she had to carry her around on a pillow to help avoid breaking her sister's fragile bones.

---

How can you tell when your child's disability has become a normal part of your family? Creating an inclusive family takes time, but there are some changes you can look for in yourself that let you know you're getting close to a new normal:

- You see how handsome your boy looks in his new suit, not his crutches or wheelchair.
- Your little girl is misbehaving and you feel free to discipline her, just as you do her able-bodied brothers and sisters.
- You call to reschedule your son's orthopedist's appointment because it conflicts with his piano recital or his sister's Little League game.
- You go out for the evening with your spouse or accept a date, leaving your children with a babysitter, and do not worry about them for the entire evening.
- You no longer ask "can" or "should" but instead "how" all your children will participate in an activity or achieve their goals.

---

"It was upsetting," Zoey says, "but she's smart. It's only physical and she can live a full life."

What's more, many sibs of kids who have disabilities are able to recognize the challenges in their own lives and have a greater appreciation that *all* people have some kind of limitations; they are part of the human condition and therefore normal. Jean observes, "Everyone has an obstacle, but it doesn't change the person's personality." Michelle O'Brien says of herself and her able-bodied sisters, "All of us have 'special needs'; they just may not be apparent on the exterior."

# PART II

## All in the Family

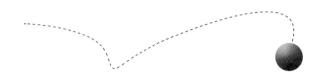

**The Bowers:** An athletic couple sort out what works for them in raising their only child, a serious student and accomplished wheelchair athlete

April and Runner married in their late twenties. "I'm in love with my husband," April beams. "I can't say enough about him." Runner agrees that their marriage is "excellent, and it's gotten even better over time. I can't see being without her." April is an occupational therapist, and Runner was a computer programmer before becoming a stay-at-home dad to Lance.

April always wanted to be a parent, but Runner "resisted having children. I didn't want to be pulled from sports and the freedom we had. We were making two good incomes. Parenting was too much responsibility."

"We were married ten years and then . . . surprise!" says April. Runner was "not happy" at the prospect of becoming a father. "But it was the best thing that ever happened to me. The instant I saw my son it was pure love, happiness; everything changed." Lance was "the perfect baby," born happy. He became the focus of their lives, even going for runs with April and Runner in the baby jogger.

When Lance was about 4, they noticed he had some bruising while they were vacationing in Florida. Doctors said it was just "growing pains," but they asked for a blood test, and then a second. The physical exam was repeated. The doctor told April that something was amiss and sent them to a hematologist. A bone marrow biopsy was done, and Lance was diagnosed with leukemia. April recalled the oncologist saying, "'It doesn't look good.' They assumed that being an OT [occupational therapist] I should know the implications."

Lance started chemotherapy. The illness went into remission, but he developed hand tremors that were a side effect of the treatment. Then, while April was at work one day, her sister called to tell her, "Lance is staggering. He can't walk." Runner remembers that when he arrived home, Lance was standing and took a few steps. Then his legs buckled. "We went to the ER."

The doctor wasn't sure if the side effects of chemotherapy were causing Lance's inability to walk—or even stand—but he suspended chemotherapy while he observed Lance's condition. At first, Lance was strong from the waist up and could propel his own wheelchair. Several weeks later he was paralyzed from the neck down and could hardly breathe. Runner wondered, "Is this how his life is going to be? When I saw Lance he smiled and said, 'Can you scratch my nose, Daddy?'"

Life was changing rapidly. For a few months Lance remained paralyzed in all four limbs. Then he slowly began to recover, and a year later he had regained his upper body strength though his legs remained paralyzed. His final diagnosis was paraplegia due to a rare neurotoxic reaction to the chemotherapy.

Each family member was affected emotionally by Lance's illness and paralysis. Going to the hospital for treatments, Lance would get angry, saying he wanted to "blow up" the hospital. April asked him about the people inside, and he would say, well, of course, he would get everyone out first.

"When Lance was going through paralysis, I couldn't stop crying," April remembers. "I went to a counselor who helped me find resources for him. She helped me see I was going through grief." April realized she wasn't crazy to have feelings of loss, anger, sadness, and frustration. April found that her "faith in God" also helped her cope during Lance's health crisis. "I prayed all the time asking God to give me strength. I feel He listened to me." One evening when Lance was in the hospital, April and Runner were in bed, crying. "Then a feeling of calm came over me. A voice said, 'Everything will be okay.' Some people lose faith when a child incurs a disability; others believe more resolutely."

Runner lost faith in Lance's doctors and hospitals. He was angry that Lance had not gone through an inpatient rehabilitation program right after he became paralyzed. After Lance's leukemia stabilized, Runner located a different hospital, which "was like a new family, seventy-five miles away. We drove there three times a week for Lance to begin a new regime of chemotherapy and to get outpatient rehabilitation."

Their families and friends were "in sync" with them, says April. Her mother, whom April thought of as her best friend, had died earlier, and she missed her. Runner says his mother was wonderful; she provided food, watched Lance, and visited in the hospital. She helped when Lance got sick, as did April's father when he flew in. Some siblings visited and supported them; others had difficulty dealing with what was happening and remained distant.

Lance needed full-time care, so April and Runner had to decide who would stay home with him. Ultimately, Runner gave up his career to be a stay-at-home dad. "I was dedicated to Lance. That helped." But it was a difficult choice for Runner and a sacrifice for all of them when their income was cut in half. April became the primary breadwinner, and they had to learn how to balance their new roles. Besides being the at-home parent, Runner does all the bill paying. April is a "clean freak" and has had to let that go. She would like to attend doctor's appointments with Lance but relies on Runner's reports.

When Lance was 8, his chemotherapy came to an end. They had a big party to celebrate. Runner was uneasy during the first year following cessation of therapy because Lance was vulnerable to a relapse. He worried about it day after day until the year passed. Then one day he realized he had gone an entire day without thinking about the possibility of relapse. "That felt good," he says.

Life in the community has not changed for them, other than their realization that "there are lots of great people." April affirms that their experience made her more thankful to people who cared about a child they didn't even know. She says she is sad that there are also folks out there with prejudice against people who have disabilities. "I would take my 4-year-old out in his wheelchair and people would stare and ask, 'What happened?'"

Lance, a teenager now, says, "When you are in a wheelchair, people judge you before they know you. It frustrates me. Once they get to know someone, then they help and are thoughtful."

An outgoing, positive wheelchair athlete, Lance is also in a unique academic high school program focusing on real-world applications of ideas. He describes himself as ambitious and serious about achievement. He is among the top-ranked hand cyclists in a competitive national circuit. He also plays wheelchair basketball competitively and travels to regional tourneys.

Although Lance has several friends at school, he tends not to socialize outside of school. He likes to spend time on his Xbox. His closest friend moved away recently, so they visit a couple of times a year. Most of his good friends are the adult wheelchair athletes with whom he travels and competes. He finds that other kids are not serious or don't care enough in school.

Risk taking is also important to Lance. "I'm a daredevil. I pop wheelies but I'm also safe." Runner says that when Lance goes biking alone, "it's worrisome because he's low to the ground and hard to see." He continually warns his son of the hazards while at the same time trying to let Lance care for himself.

A typical teen, Lance doesn't pick up his room as his parents would like him to—although he feels he helps out a lot, clearing the dinner table, setting out silverware, and keeping his bathroom clean. April and Runner feel they haven't given him enough responsibility and do too much for him. And they also have some concerns about their lack of consistency in enforcing rules or limits for Lance.

As for the future, Lance says he will study aeronautical engineering. He loves airplanes and admires his father's engineering mind. He might also become a professional hand cyclist. He asserts, "Having a disability doesn't mean you can't do anything. You have to find a reason for life and have a positive outlook. Because I was injured so young, disability shaped my outlook and the way I was going to be. I don't take life for granted."

Runner notes, "We search out opportunities to get our son involved in. We want him to participate in basketball and hand cycling. It has shaped all of our lives." He and Lance also do adaptive skiing together. He advises families not to withdraw and close in on themselves, but instead to seek new opportunities for themselves as a family and for their child who has a disability. He and April can see that the many trips Lance has taken with his basketball team have helped him mature and become even more independent.

April has found that "patience with your spouse and yourself helps" with parenting. She has learned not to worry about the little things and become more caring of herself and her family. She agrees with Runner that looking for the best resources is imperative when you have a child who has a physical disability.

# 3

# Inclusive Parenting

**Make It Work for You**

------------------------------------------------------------------------

"Being a parent has given me more to live for, more to appreciate about life. I look at the world with a sense of purpose. Having a child has an impact; having a child who has a physical disability has an even greater impact. I can't separate the two. It's a lot more work, but rewarding. I have to be positive and tough in a way. I have a lot more love than I knew I had."

> —KATHLEEN, MOTHER OF
> A SON WHO HAS SPINA
> BIFIDA

In this chapter we look first at how you can *take care of yourself*, so you can be a more effective parent, and secondly at how you can *build resilience in your kids*. Taking care of yourself means getting enough support (from your partner, family, and friends), finding ways to cope with your emotions, setting priorities and letting go of unnecessary tasks, taking time out for yourself, and learning from experienced parents. Building resilience in your kids involves creating expectations for success, giving them responsibilities, allowing some risk taking, enriching their life experiences, and boosting their self-esteem by being a positive role model.

## First Things First: Get Support for Parenting

All parents need to support their children economically (usually by working outside the home), create a safe and secure home, and supply the nurturance, education, and love necessary for their kids to thrive. Each family divides these jobs in different ways. But no matter how you slice it, parenting is one tough job! You need support from other adults to be the best parent you can be.

## Support from Your Partner

If you are part of a couple—mom and dad, two moms, two dads, or a parent and stepparent—you support each other, make decisions as a team, and share the task of building an inclusive family.

### Working as a Team

When your child is born with or develops a physical disability, having a strong, intimate tie with your partner can help you with parenting. Rose found that learning to confide in her husband and becoming his "best friend" was essential to her parenting success. Paul, the father of twins, one of whom was born with a disability, found that "working as a team" helped him and his wife cope with stress and solve problems. April and Runner, whose son Lance has a spinal cord injury, agree. "We relied on and appreciated one another, and Lance's illness brought us closer," says Runner. Their support for each other sets the tone for the family; "I think it's good for Lance to see how we feel about each other," says April.

D. K. and his wife have a "very good, understanding relationship. We are strong spouses for each other. We are both strong willed, perseverance based, and have a no-quitting attitude. We make our marriage and family work and do not compromise the lives of our children."

In short, support and teamwork strengthen a couple's partnership—and also help them take better care of their kids. Some parents worry that time spent with each other will mean less time for their kids or less effective parenting. But actually, nurturing your relationship with your partner makes you a better parent.

### Keeping an Intimate Connection

Parenting seems all-encompassing at times, threatening to crowd out your intimate emotional and sexual life as a couple. Setting aside some time each day to talk with your partner without the kids around, going on "dates," and getting away for a weekend now and then are some ways to avoid losing this vital connection with your partner. Scheduling time for your sexual relationship can also be helpful, as privacy is scarce during the day, and after the kids are asleep one or both of you may be too tired. Getting some extra help with the kids a couple of days a week can leave you more energy for making love on those nights. On other nights, cuddling with your partner before going to sleep can help you feel closer and more relaxed and encourage sharing of intimate emotions. When you feel loved and supported by your partner, you are better able to cope with stress and can bring renewed enthusiasm to parenting.

## Support from Other Sources

### Grandparents Can Help

Even if you and your partner work smoothly as a parenting team, there are times when both of you run out of energy and need a break to recharge. Getting away from home for a few days is incredibly restorative. Grandparents (or other relatives) can really help, especially when your child has extensive care needs, by caring for your children while you are gone.

Kathleen's son has spina bifida, and there are few babysitters who can handle his needs, but Kathleen's mother has learned to manage his complex care. She stays with her grandson several weekends a year so Kathleen can go away with her husband. Last year she stayed with him for ten days while Kathleen and her husband went on an extended vacation. These special times with her husband help Kathleen enjoy and nurture her marriage, unwind, and gather energy for the next phase of parenting.

### Community Resources Can Back You Up

Even if your family members can't take care of your child who has a physical disability, there are other options in the community, including short-term residential services or week-long or weekend camping experiences. These programs, sometimes called respite care, allow parents to get away for a few days, knowing that their child is with experienced caregivers. Many private home care agencies employ trained people who can stay with your child for a few days or a few hours. These services range

Sleepaway summer camps for kids who have disabilities offer sessions of one or more weeks, allowing you and your spouse a much-needed break while providing fun and stimulating activities for your child. Look for camps in the Resources section of this book.

from babysitters to certified nursing assistants to registered nurses, depending on your child's needs.

## Support for Single Parents

If you are a single parent of a child who has a disability, the support of other adults—family, friends, or hired helpers—is critical to your success, as well as your sanity! When you don't have a partner, you are "it"—the teacher, cheerleader, decision maker, consoler, goal setter, and disciplinarian for your children. Finding support from other adults is one of the secrets to success as a single parent. Some single parents exchange nights of babysitting for each other's kids so each can have some free time. "Bartering" with friends to meet each other's needs is another approach. For instance, Dorothy, an excellent seamstress, often hems a skirt or makes a dress for her friend's daughter, in exchange for her friend's babysitting services.

Susie's experience illustrates how challenging single parenting can be when your family includes children who have physical disabilities—and how, with support, you can do it.

Susie was married and a working mother of four little boys, including twins with a muscle disorder. When her twins were 17 months old, her husband suddenly decided to leave the family. Susie prayed for guidance and believed that God was telling her, "It's not going to work out but you can manage it." In time she "learned that I was stronger than I knew."

After her separation, Susie had no health insurance for herself and her boys. The twins had not yet been formally diagnosed, but they had abnormal muscle tone and weakness. Their condition fluctuated; at one point Susie was told they might die. As babies they had no strength in their necks so their heads needed extra support. One twin had curvature of the spine, and both were delayed in their physical development. Finally, the boys were diagnosed with benign congenital hypotonia and sent to a specialty hospital for treatment. Susie was working part-time and spending two to three hours a day doing physical therapy with the twins. Besides this daily exercise regimen, Susie had to carry the boys when they were sick or when they had used up their limited energy and were too exhausted to walk. Fortunately, she discovered the Mothers of Twins Club, and they helped her out one afternoon a week for several years.

When her husband walked out, Susie was left alone to deal with four of life's biggest stress factors: the birth of a baby (× 2!), disability, the breakup of a marriage, and loss of health insurance for the family. Susie could not do it all alone—and discovered that she didn't have to. She found the emotional and practical support she needed from her family, friends, and volunteers. Susie also coped exceptionally well with this crisis by drawing on her inner strengths and the social values passed down from her parents. With the "hard work" ethic and expectations for success instilled by her own family, Susie had guideposts to follow for raising her children and for continuing to live productively in other ways.

Mia is another single mother of four children, the youngest with osteogenesis imperfecta (OI). After many years of marriage, she divorced her husband, who was an alcoholic and an unreliable father. Mia has to support her family by working full-time plus teaching two nights a week. Although there are downsides—especially the few hours of sleep each night!—she takes pride in the way the family works. They are highly organized, with a schedule of chores for everyone to contribute to running the household. Mia also makes sure that the kids have time to play with friends and do the things they love to do. She brings an upbeat sense of humor to mothering; she likes to "get crazy and play jokes on the kids" to lighten the tone in the family. While Mia's children do not have the benefits of a second parent in the house, Mia feels proud of her resilience as a parent who is able to provide economically for her kids and to nurture and guide them.

Blake is a single father of George, a teenager who has a spinal cord injury. His wife left the family when George was 6. Blake reorganized his life, going from his traveling sales job to a predictable nine-to-five job with good insurance benefits close to home. Blake's sister helped him out by watching George after school until Blake got home from work. After George's injury, at 13, Blake's sister learned how to take care of him, so Blake could get away for a weekend once in a while. As a solo parent of a teen who's campaigning for his independence, Blake has to work a little harder to maintain his role as the family decision maker. But he talks openly with George about problems and takes his opinions seriously. Currently, Blake is weighing George's need to be independent, i.e., drive a car, with concern for his son's safety. They have resolved the problem by scheduling frequent cell phone check-ins (while parked) when George is out with the car.

As Blake and Susie found, extended family can be a vital source of support for single parents, ranging from phone or e-mail check-ins, to dinners or overnight visits, to financial help. Even if they can't provide practical or economic assistance, your family's respect and regard for the job you are doing are very helpful. Let them know when you need some encouragement and approval. When your family's ability to help is limited, friends can be a valuable backup. Members of your religious congregation, parent-teacher association, or community center may offer emotional support or child care while you get some rest. If you are a single mom with sons or a single dad with daughters, you may be able to find a same-sex role model and mentor for your child through the Big Brothers Big Sisters organization in your town.

## Step Two: Coping with Your Emotions

Before you can tackle any new job, you need to "clear the decks." Difficult emotions sap your energy and limit your ability to focus on finding solutions. You need to identify and cope with emotional reactions to your child's disability before you can move on to learning about your child's needs and solving problems.

Parents have different approaches to coping with emotions. Some parents need to "let it all out," while others work through their emotional reactions internally. This can be a brief or lengthy process. Priscilla found that just having a good cry after learning that her child would have spina bifida brought relief—enough that she could begin the search for information to educate herself and her husband about this condition. Kathleen allows herself a fifteen-minute "freak-out" when she's "had it" emotionally. She takes a quick run around the block, and the physical exercise gets her off the emotional roller coaster and helps her clarify the problem and find solutions. Mark finds that writing about disturbing feelings and looking for triggers that "set him off" help him understand his emotions and regain composure. Then he's in "a better space" to explore solutions.

Other parents find that working out solutions is, in itself, a way to cope with their feelings about a problem. These parents spring into action from the start, dealing with hurt, anger, or sadness by *doing something*— such as seeking the advice of experts, surfing the Internet for information, building a ramp for a child who uses a wheelchair, or doing some other task that will solve a practical problem for their child or family. Sometimes taking the first step to tackle a problem helps you feel more in control of your life, which can make you feel calmer.

## Step Three: Taking Care of Yourself

As a parent, you need to keep a balance between your family's needs and your own; you need to take care of *yourself*, not just your kids! Parents often sacrifice for their kids, neglecting themselves in the bargain. But this can backfire, because if you become ill, exhausted, or emotionally burned out, your parenting will take a nosedive. "Maintain" yourself and your physical and mental health by getting medical checkups, exercising, relaxing, and having some fun.

### Take a Time-out

One way to manage the stress of parenting is to take a time-out to focus on what *you* need. Periodic getaways can give you a reprieve from the daily grind. Make sure you don't wait to take a break until you've reached the point of exhaustion! A time-out is not just a chance to collapse, but rather time to kick back and relax, to enjoy your friends, hobbies, or leisure pursuits—and to relish life apart from your role as a parent.

If you have a partner, friend, or other supportive person in your life, they can remind you to take a break and be there to back you up. Evelyn's husband, Scott, is a loving stepdad to her daughter Celeste, who has OI. Evelyn makes sure to take regular "downtimes" for rest and relaxation, free of her usual responsibilities. "I take care of myself so that I can be a better, whole, capable person to care for the kids. Scott's job," she says,

*Mom's or Dad's time-out.* Important for all parents, especially single parents, is a "time-out"—perhaps a movie with friends; a long, relaxing bath; a one-mile run; or ten minutes of sitting in the sun. The important thing is that it's just for you and makes you feel good. This is one of the tricks of a resilient parent—knowing how to create a bit of peace or enjoyment to restoke energy.

T Watch your sense of balance. Are you taking good care of yourself?
Ask yourself if you've had enough fun lately. Have you been tickled by the absurd recently? Have you laughed out loud? Did you see the brilliance of last evening's sunset? Have you heard any good music lately? When did you last feel completely relaxed? If you can't remember the last time you enjoyed one of these "simple pleasures," you need to make more time for yourself!

"is to care for *me* so that I can do that. It makes a big difference in the kids' lives."

Experienced parents agree that it's important *not* to define yourself solely through your role as a mother or father. Maintaining an identity as an individual contributes to good mental health. There are many ways to do this. Many parents find meaning in getting together with friends, doing volunteer work, joining a book club, or taking a class. Runner loves to read for relaxation and enjoyment. "I go to the library once a week." Lee enjoys shooting and hunting, while other fathers enjoy running or woodworking. When you do things that make you feel good about yourself and the world, you have more energy to engage and be creative with your children.

## Take Charge of Your Schedule

"There just aren't enough hours in the day!" is the universal mantra of busy parents. If this is true for most parents, how do those with a child who has a physical disability manage to fit in the needs of the whole family? Susie carved out time in her schedule to fit in her twins' exercise regime while continuing as a volunteer in programs for her two older sons. Since it was impossible to do it all at one time, Susie focused on one of the boys per year, alternating years of being a room mother for the oldest boy with leading her second son's Cub Scout den. Wisely, Susie realized she needed to set some limits on her time in order to protect her health, essential to mothering all her boys.

For many parents, there are times when the needs of their children are greater than they can manage. Both Larry and Pili experienced the time crunch that a child's physical disability adds to the family routine. Larry remembers the frequent feedings his son needed in the first year of life, the nights when he and his wife slept in shifts, and the amount of extra time and energy he spent with his son during his many surgeries. Pili's schedule includes catheterizing her child every few hours plus the extra time it takes to prepare equipment they need for trips outside the home. Liz, a single working parent, agrees that the biggest difference having a child who has a physical disability made in her family life was the need for more time, given the daily routine of dressing and changing her daughter, putting on her braces, chauffeuring her, and trying to meet her son's needs.

For most parents, these times of being overwhelmed by too much to do are temporary, and they can muddle through by putting some non-parenting responsibilities on the back burner. In those families where there's no letup, you need to find additional help or support. Often, the time demands ease as children get older and more independent.

Parents find that, by prioritizing the needs of their family, they can make time stretch. Mary found that with her daughter's disability everything took more time, and life seemed to be moving in "slow motion." But this slower pace had a positive side, too, allowing Mary to really listen and take a good look at what was happening in her family. She didn't want to let the time needed for physical disability–related needs trump activities that each of her other children found fulfilling. But something had to give to make it work. Mary's solution was to figure out which activities were either absolutely necessary or uplifting to the life of the family and to eliminate those activities that weren't. She reset her expectations about what she *had* to do, putting all the unessential tasks in the "optional" column and setting aside certain home chores and projects. Letting go of that perfectionist "getting it all done" mind-set can help you find the time not only for the necessities of life but for the activities that your children—and you—are passionate about and find energizing. Runner and his wife found that parenting their son who has a spinal cord injury was overwhelming with both parents working outside the home. Although Runner always thought he *had* to work, he and his wife agreed that Lance was their priority; ultimately Runner chose to leave his job so he could be there whenever Lance needed him. Though their income "was cut in half," Runner has no regrets. "I like my time with Lance, and this gives all of us a great family life."

Interestingly, some parents find that during their busiest times they are highly efficient and actually get more things accomplished, taking on projects they have not done before. Charlotte, for instance, planted an enormous flower and vegetable garden while she had two toddlers at home and her daughter was going through a series of spinal operations. As the old saying goes, "If you want to get something done, ask a busy person to do it." While some parents benefit from letting go of nonessential activities, others with excessive demands on their time can cope by relying on a high degree of organization and multitasking—and sometimes manage so well that there is time "left over" to take a breather. Sometimes extra activities, like working in the garden, are pleasurable and renewing, making it easier to manage those things that weigh you down. Creating projects that you plan for and control can help you cope better with the unexpected and uncontrollable demands and challenges of life.

## Find Friends

Parents who seem to "have it together," able to manage their families under challenging circumstances, are often people who have supportive friends. Friendships improve parents' self-esteem, provide practical help and emotional support, and add meaning to parents' lives.

We all add and subtract friends during different phases in our lives. Parents lose some when their children are born with or develop disabilities; certain friends can't cope with the idea of disability and seem awkward and unsure about what to ask, how to be helpful, or how to interact with your child. Cindy found that friends had trouble both at the time of her son's birth and later, when he had to have treatments. "When people find out about Xavier, they use the typical sayings, phrases like 'hang in there' or 'everything happens for a reason.' Some of the sayings helped when they were sincere. But the best thing anyone did for me was to be there, just sit with me at the hospital, or eat lunch or dinner with me. They really didn't have to say much; just being there was a great support in itself." It's important to find a friend who can listen and try to understand your experience, without judging or trying to change your feelings. This sort of empathy ("I'm in it with you") is a special kind of support that is essential for your emotional balance. Friends can also help with things like babysitting or going to the grocery store for you. You may need to rely on different friends for each of these two types of support—being with or doing things for you. You can also let your friends know which type of support you need (and your needs will be different at different times), for example, by saying, "You know, I don't really need you to *do* anything right now, but if you can just spend time talking with me, listening to me, that would help me so much!" Or alternatively, "I really need to rest today—I'm too tired to even talk. Could you possibly pick up some milk and cereal for me while I get a nap?"

All parents need emotional support from friends and peers, but mothers and fathers of kids who have disabilities need an extra dollop. Men tend to have fewer close friendships than their wives, and many feel alone when coping with the initial diagnosis of a child's disability and during the months or years in which parenting requires the largest share of their time and energy. When you are a new parent, or one whose child has just acquired a physical disability, it's helpful to make new friends with whom you can bond over your common experiences as parents. You will find that many parents are accepting of children who have disabilities and see this as just another individual variation—even if their own children do not have disabilities. Claude felt unsure about how his son—or he himself—would be accepted into a scouting troop. He was pleased when the leader integrated his son into a variety of activities and invited Claude to take a central role in planning. Not only did Claude and the troop leader become close friends, but involvement with the scouts opened up friendships with other fathers who were helping the troop. A key for parents is not to assume that others will have a negative view of your child or the role of disability in your lives. Many families are eager to integrate children with all sorts of unique experiences and backgrounds into their own children's friendships, including kids who have physical disabilities. Parents are wise to assume the positive until proved otherwise, taking the risk to help your child initiate relationships with a variety of people. Although some will not be interested, many will.

### Learn from Parents Who Know the Ropes

Being friends with parents whose children don't have disabilities can help you (and your child) keep disability in perspective and lessen your feelings of "other-ness." But it's also helpful to get support and learn from

other parents of kids who have disabilities. As Pili says, "It's incredible to
share your journey with parents of kids who have other disabilities," not
only the same disability that your child has. "It's good to have someone
you can connect with." Throughout the various stages of your family life,
you can benefit from the expertise and advice of parents who have "been
there." Having a mentoring relationship, where you can learn one-on-one
from a more experienced mother or father, is invaluable.

## Building Resilience
### Meet Every Child's Needs

"How can I ever meet all their needs?" "How can I make sure each
child gets a fair share of my time and attention?" While balancing the
needs of each family member is a challenge for every parent, making sure
that basics are met is the first priority. Beyond that, parents need to create
ways to pay attention to each child, as well as sharing family time. Lola
and her husband make a routine of giving their undivided attention to
each child whenever he or she has a special event or has accomplished a
new goal. For instance, when their older son makes honor roll at school,
they celebrate with him; the following week their middle son basks in the
limelight at a chess tournament; and their daughter has the focus when
she dances in a recital. Extra care and attention are also given to family
members when they have extra needs—like when their son needed surgery or when Lola underwent treatment for cancer. Philip and Lola got
help from their extended families during these crises, so they could pro-

vide extra support to the family member who was hospitalized, while continuing to pay attention to the other children.

Liz has been more concerned at times about the development of her able-bodied son than her daughter who has a disability. She advises other parents to give special time to their able-bodied kids, too.

Liz's busy work schedule meant that often the needs of her daughter who has spina bifida took first priority. But when Liz had sabbaticals from teaching, she took the children abroad with her. During these trips, she had more time than usual to participate in activities with her kids, to listen to and talk with them, and to focus specifically on the needs and desires of her son who does not have a disability. These sabbaticals also gave Liz's children exposure to different cultures and the opportunity to visit historical sites.

Some parents emphasize family unity more than individual relationships between each child and parent. They express inclusiveness by finding ways for their child who has a disability to be a part of shared family vacations and leisure activities and by making sure she plays a meaningful role in how the family works. Lee, for example, takes his family to an accessible beach camp in the summer, where all the children can participate in outdoor activities. Scott likes to bring the whole family together for Sunday brunches, where everyone goofs off and jokes, creating "a veritable laugh riot." He believes that family outings and activities that include all the children create a "more enriched experience" and are vital to family closeness. He's not against doing things individually with one child, but he notes that in his family "if you split up the kids, they wish everyone was doing something together."

After her daughter's accident, Marie worked hard to create family solidarity and avoid sibling rivalry by having big family dinners in the tradition of her Italian parents. "We sit around the table as a family and share the day. Everyone has a chance to talk and communicate." While a sense of family togetherness is emphasized and strengthened by these dinners, Marie and her husband try to make sure that each member of the family is also individually recognized and listened to.

In D. K.'s family, most of the leisure activities are on the water, where everyone can join in. Swimming is relatively safe for Dan (who has OI)

> "Look out for the well-being of your children without a disability. Give them time, listen to their emotions. Be mindful of them." —Liz

and enjoyed by all the kids. D. K. jokes that he and his wife "created a family of good swimmers" by putting in an Endless Pool. They value boating, because it, too, "keeps the family intact." Once in a while, they split up the family for special outings; D. K. might take Dan to a museum while his wife, Erica, takes their two able-bodied children skiing.

It can be particularly challenging for parents to pay attention to the needs of all children when one has a medical problem or is in the hospital. Advanced preparation for these crises is very helpful. For example, Erica keeps ready a grab bag of games, toys, books, and little gifts for the times when Dan breaks a bone and the recuperation periods that follow. Other parents prepare fun activities ahead of time, such as DVDs and new computer games, which can be shared by the child who is recuperating and his siblings—who are likely to be more limited to home-based activities when their brother or sister is ill.

## Expect Success

There are many ways to help your kids learn how to care for themselves and respect the needs of others at the same time. Methods need to be tailored to each child's personality strengths and weaknesses. Some children are self-driven and goal oriented. They may be prone to overreach and feel defeated. Jasmine, a high school student, has rheumatoid arthritis. She is a straight A student taking several honors classes. When she does not meet her self-imposed goals, she becomes overly critical of herself. Her parents try to help her ease up on the high expectations she has for herself. They remind her that they love her for who she is as a person, and that her accomplishments are just icing on the cake. When they think she is overloading herself, they try to "rein her in" by making suggestions for lightening her course load. They help her balance her load so that she can be successful.

Other kids need to be motivated and pushed a bit. Gerald is happy playing computer games and hanging out with his friends, but he has little interest in schoolwork. His parents set up incentives for him (working to get an iPad) to complete his school assignments and disincentives (loss of computer time) for goofing off. They help him through feelings of inferiority that sometimes interfere with his trying to do his best.

Carmen's 7-year-old daughter, Mercedes, home after treatment for a traumatic automobile accident, had grown accustomed to being waited on in the hospital. She began to think that her disability entitled her to special consideration—forever! Back home, however, she had older and younger sisters who had needs of their own. One day she threw a tantrum when she didn't get the Lego kit she wanted at the toy store. Carmen realized that it was time to fit her daughter back into the family system by saying "No" and giving her some responsibilities. She began a "respectful love" regimen with her daughter. Carmen set higher expectations for her daughter's behavior, letting Mercedes know that she respected and believed in her abilities. Soon Mercedes was working in the kitchen in her wheelchair, drying the silverware and putting it in the drawer. This was the beginning of her preparation for independence through developing competency and thinking of others.

Some children find controlling their emotions and behavior difficult and need extra help in changing it. Skip was disruptive at school and alienating friends and family with his outlandish behaviors. His parents had him tested by a psychologist, who diagnosed his problem as attention deficit disorder, manageable with medication and therapy. With this support, his grades are slowly improving and he has started to make some new friends.

## Teach Responsibility

Teaching your child that she has obligations to herself and others is a major goal of parenting. How do you teach that we all have duties to our fellow human beings, particularly our parents and siblings? When we hear about "spoiled" children, we are really hearing about children who have not been taught how to think of and do for others. Shaping a child to be responsible begins early in the child's life, and this job rests with the parent.

In most families, parents decide together how chores or responsibilities will be assigned to their children, but often one parent is the "heavy" while the other is the "softie" when it comes to discipline and follow-through. Sean, for instance, would like to demand more from his kids, while his wife, Leigh, he feels, is more likely to be "manipulated" and let the kids slide on their chores. On the other hand, they both enforce high standards of academic achievement and expect commitment from their girls to practice piano and go out for sports. Leigh feels that those standards require time and effort and that home chores rank low on the priority list.

Finding the right combination of love and discipline can be a process of trial and error. Carson believes that consistent but loving discipline is the key to raising responsible children. Part of being an inclusive parent is applying the same standards of behavior (politeness, honesty, timely completion of schoolwork, and so forth) to his son, Brian, who has a severe physical disability, and to his able-bodied daughter, Cory. Carson notes that good discipline leads to good behavior, and he hopes that good behavior will lead to acceptance, respect, and love for Brian from those outside the family circle. This will be essential to Brian's survival, understanding of give and take, and enjoyment of life when he is living away from the family as a young adult.

## Let Your Kids Take Some Risks

Parents expose their kids to life experiences that can broaden their child's physical and mental skills, knowledge, creativity, and character. Risk taking is often part and parcel of these experiences. Children learn through trying new activities and relationships and by making (and correcting) mistakes. For example, taking the risk to expand a circle of friends exposes them to rejection, while participating in physical activities strengthens their bodies but also includes the risk of injury.

Parents often hesitate when their kids take risks to expand their worlds with new friends, activities, or sports. This anxiety is doubled when your son or daughter has a physical disability. After the initial attempts at some new activity, your concern is usually overcome when you meet your child's new friends, see him up on stage in the school play, or watch him make his first hit in the Little League game. You will discover that a good experience in one area will increase your (and your child's) openness to other "risks" in different areas.

The support of other adults who interact with your children can help you encourage risk taking and new experiences. Runner's son Lance plays wheelchair basketball, and the first time Lance traveled with his team, Runner was nervous. But Lance's coach told him, "We'll take care of him." Lance has since traveled nationally and internationally; now that Runner knows that Lance can take care of himself on the road, he tries to find other opportunities that will help Lance increase his physical and social independence. The first step in "letting go" is always the hardest.

If you are worried about your child spreading his wings, discussing your fears with your partner, your parents, or another trusted adult can help you assess your child's readiness to take reasonable risks. If your partner also has a disability, she may be more comfortable with risk taking and be able to give you a unique perspective. Jalah and her son Jon both have OI. Jon recalls that it was "harder on Dad" to let him take risks, "harder for him to see me get hurt," while it was "less hard for Mom because she grew up with it." Jalah's confidence in her own abilities provided a role model that encouraged reasonable risks, balancing her husband's tendency to be protective. Jalah advises parents to "let your child set their own limits and not feel sorry for the child because this can cripple them. Let them be who they can be and do what they can do."

Julius emphasizes the importance of helping children with their fears when it comes to risk taking. He knows that his daughter must take some risks to fully enjoy life and gain competence. "You can't ignore your child's fears, but you have to help her focus on what she can do, not what she can't." Julius encouraged his daughter, who lost a leg in an accident, to try out for wheelchair track events in high school. She loved it and became a regular competitor in college. "That's what a little confidence can do for you," Julius says proudly.

> "I don't want my daughter to be held back by her disability and afraid of living. I want her to say, 'That's what I want,' and go for it." —Julius

Broad-mindedness and flexibility help parents find novel activities that expand their children's world of skills and experiences but are not beyond their physical limits. One mother encouraged her son to take a modern dance class when he couldn't "make the cut" for any of his school's team sports. At first her son, a 15-year-old with a muscle disorder, was mortified, but when he realized he'd be getting a great workout—and exercising with a lot of girls wearing tights—he became an enthusiastic dancer.

As your child who has a physical disability matures, he becomes increasingly able to judge his own abilities and limitations; he can collaborate with you in making decisions about risk taking. You can talk directly with him to weigh the pros and cons of various risks—the possibility of

> **T**Children have dreams of what they'll do in life, whether it's going to the moon, being an NBA star forward, or becoming a firefighter. Parents listen to these dreams and set no limits on this imagination. However, when your daughter who walks with braces and crutches dreams of being a prima ballerina, you may want to step in to redirect that dream to protect her from future disappointment. Restrain yourself! Step back as you do with your other children, allowing your daughter to make her own personal discovery of what she is able to do, in her own time.

hurt or disappointment versus the chance to have a special experience or accomplish a new goal. Felicity, a young woman who has a spinal cord injury, advises parents not to "judge the abilities of your child who has a disability." Although parents try to empathize with their child's experience, Felicity says that "they don't really know what the child is going through." She urges parents to let their child try to do the things he or she wants to do, because kids who have physical disabilities are stronger and wiser than others might think. Sometimes, what we think is impossible isn't. Billy had both legs amputated below the knee; he loved baseball and became a star pitcher on his high school team, even running bases without prostheses.

Jon agrees that parents don't always appreciate the strengths of their child who has a disability. He feels that the child should be "a large part of the decision making team" regarding when to let the child take certain risks. Jon's parents let him take a major role in judging risks, and he notes, "I was pretty intuitive about knowing what would hurt." Because he has OI, some bone breaks were inevitable—regardless of Jon's level of risk taking. Jon believes that even the extra breaks were worthwhile experiences—they made him more resilient and determined. "I can stick with something because I had to keep getting back up. It's hard to defeat me."

## Boost Self-Esteem with Positive Role Modeling

All kids—whether or not they have disabilities—look to their parents as the keys to creating a positive self-image and self-esteem. For kids who have disabilities, resiliency depends in part on learning to value their own

Parents need to continually weigh the risks and benefits of a child who has a disability joining in activities with siblings or friends. If your child has arm strength but not leg strength, she can bike using a three-wheeled, hand-propelled bike, or sail down a mountainside on a sit-ski, tethered to an able-bodied skier. Even with adaptations, the risks involved in sledding or horseback riding, especially for a child with OI, must be considered along with the benefits to your child: should you err on the side of "staying safe" or risk a little to enhance your child's life experience?

talents, character traits, and abilities, rather than basing their self-worth on how their bodies look or work. Be open to discussing this if your child is grappling with the way he thinks others see him. For example, listen when your child brings up the unfairness of having physical limitations and how hard it is to feel excluded when other kids are playing sports. Tell her she has a right to her feelings and repeat those feelings back to her, so she knows you are really hearing her. When she has finished, remind her of her talents, her abilities, and what is available to her. And reassure your son that he is loved for himself, not his linebacker abilities. Once again, the importance of keeping balanced in life emerges; when your child feels pulled down, you can help him counterbalance by talking about and exposing him to uplifting activities and experiences. Remind her that many other opportunities will come along as she gets older and then the things that are so important now—like running and playing soccer—will not be as important.

Beatrice Wright, one of the first psychologists to examine the psychological experience of living with disability, notes that individuals who have physical disabilities develop a positive sense of self by making changes in their values; rather than measuring their worth through physical prowess, they learn to value their personal attributes—such as intelligence, warmth, humor, and so forth. They focus on what they can rather than can't do, and they evaluate goals more in terms of the ends (can they get the job done?) than the means (did they have to use a brace or walker to do it?).

Parents of children who have disabilities go through a parallel change in values, leading to a different way of defining their own "success" as parents. Many parents measure their own worth by their children's mile-

## Confronting Stereotypes

As a parent you will need to help your child deal with the injustice of other people's preconceived notions, stereotypes, and negative attitudes about disability. Even if your child who has a physical disability is as accomplished as—or more accomplished than—an able-bodied peer, others may not believe he is capable and may perceive him as being "given" recognition or rewards out of pity. For instance, when Cory was presented the top academic award in his school, his mother heard someone say, "Oh, how nice that they gave that child the award." Clearly this person did not see Cory as achieving the honor on his own merits. Parents can help by allowing their child to talk about his anger, listening to him, and letting him know that his emotions (and their own) are justified in these situations. Then they can guide their children to recognize stereotypes without accepting them as reality. Children can use the fuel of their anger to challenge negative views and to move beyond them, so they don't become barriers. In truth, there are also many people who don't see disability at all and who focus on your child as a person.

stones in physical development, achievements in sports, or attaining conventional social goals like driving a car and going to sleepaway camp. But after raising a child who has a physical disability, parents learn to rate their "job performance" by their child's social, emotional, and moral development, the quality of his relationships with other people, and his personal characteristics—like courage, affection, or generosity. This can "rub off" on parents, changing their *self*-evaluation to one based less on their vocational and financial achievements and more on their fulfillment in how they contribute to the world's good, maintain relationships, and follow their passions.

For young children, playtime is an opportunity to develop confidence and self-esteem, especially when a parent shares their special project or hobby. Adam, a 9-year-old who has a spinal cord injury, built an entire Lego city with his father in their dining room. He felt a sense of accomplishment and pride when his father praised his imagination and skill. And from watching his dad's step-by-step approach, Adam learned that patience and care, as well as inspiration, are important to the success of a creative project.

Parents can model attitudes, emotions, and behaviors that help their children learn to manage their feelings, behave appropriately in a variety of situations, and cope with life's challenges. Kaylee, whose son, Tony, has multiple disabilities, models humor and an upbeat outlook for coping with stress. "My positive attitude's rubbed off on him. I'll say, 'Stop complaining and get on with life.' I was brought up to laugh off my troubles, and I try to pass that on. Even when Tony's sick, he'll still give me a grin and laugh at my silly jokes. He'll usually make a few of his own, too." Kaylee is quick to add, however, that she takes Tony's feelings seriously when he is having a rough time—and does not *expect* him to always be "Mr. Upbeat."

For older kids, parents can also serve as role models for academic success and be influential in their kid's career choices. Fifteen-year-old Lance, for example, admires his father's quick mind and his knowledge of electronics and software. Like his "computer whiz" dad, Lance loves technology and wants to be an engineer someday.

When a parent has a physical disability, too, his child who has a disability may have a unique learning opportunity. Raul, a young man with juvenile arthritis, says his father is "my inspiration. Dad had a nerve injury that crippled his arms, but I've never looked at him as being different." Emma, a young woman who has spina bifida, is now a mother herself. Her father has multiple sclerosis, and as she grew up, he worked hard to "desensitize me to the ridicule of peers." Jalah, who has OI, says it was "harder letting my son with OI be independent and seeing him break a bone than letting myself do the same thing. I was more protective of him" than her mother had been of Jalah.

## Reaping the Rewards of Parenting

Many parents feel unprepared for parenthood and wonder whether they are up to the task. The arrival of a new baby who has a disability can cause additional feelings of helplessness. Still, most parents "fall in love" with their newborns, whether or not they have a disability. Runner recalls that, despite his trepidation about becoming a father, Lance's birth was the "best thing that ever happened to me. The instant I saw my son it was pure love, happiness; everything changed." Later, when Lance was treated for cancer and developed a spinal cord injury, Runner found enormous satisfaction in watching him recover, grow, and develop into a lively and talented teenager.

Parents of kids who have physical disabilities experience many emotional rewards. Parenting can lead to positive personality changes or a heightened sense of purpose. Sean says that raising his daughter Eliza, who has cerebral palsy (CP), "made me more empathetic; it humanized me. I'm still a type A, but now I'm more patient." Sean has a rewarding relationship with Eliza. "I like the feedback from Eliza—when she asks me for a hug—when I see how well she is doing in college." Father to three younger daughters in addition to Eliza, Sean says that parenting is "humbling because you realize your own inadequacies. But life is more interesting with kids than without them. It sucks to get up at 6:40 on Saturday morning to line the soccer field before the game, but then you drive home with your child and say, 'Fun game, wasn't it?' "

Debbie found that caring for her son Daniel, who has a disabling joint disorder, improved her relationships with her other two children— and helped her change for the better. "I'm so much more tuned in to *each* child, what they need and their unique personalities. Daniel was the 'baby,' and before him, the older kids never really saw me express emotions. I never yelled, but I wasn't a real fun mom either. My brain was always at work or worrying about the house. With Daniel, I had to *be there*—and now I've learned how to do that with all of them. I'm a better parent because of it."

> "I wouldn't have changed a thing. Wylie's disability made me a better person." —Lee

## Creating *Your* Unique Family

Like many parents, you may have tried to fit in with the neighborhood's standard of "normal" family life. But when your child has a physical disability, these standards may not be a perfect fit. If you listen to your own inner radar and challenge social stereotypes, you can arrive at your own definition of success. When you stop worrying about the guidelines set by others, you are free to decide what works for *your child or family*. You can create a "different kind of normal" that allows every member of your family to thrive. When you believe that *all* of your children can live meaningful lives and allow yourself to do what is necessary to promote their success, you create a unique way of being an inclusive family—the way that works best for *you*.

☞ Here are some tips for making inclusive parenting work for you:

- Become educated about your child's needs. With greater knowledge and experience, your confidence in your own judgments and decisions increases, and you become proactive, not reactive.
- When you feel overwhelmed, reach out to veteran parents. You can learn from their experience and get support from them.
- Parents who find someone with whom they can share their load—whether spouse, significant other, partner, another relative, or friend—have an easier time with parenting. Multigenerational families can help share the load of raising children.
- Making the time to ensure that you feel fulfilled in your intimate life with your partner or spouse gives you more energy to bring to parenting.
- You will make the best decisions and ensure the best care for your child by partnering with professionals—physicians, physical therapists, occupational therapists, nurses, psychologists, social workers, rehabilitation counselors—in your child's treatment.
- Finding activities that give you "breathing room" outside the family is essential to restoking your energies and caring for yourself as a parent.
- Parents can help prepare their children for adulthood by giving them responsibilities to build competence, social skills to engage in relationships, experiences to understand the world, and permission to take risks so they can learn to evaluate their capabilities and what is safe and acceptable for them.
- To build resilient families, parents must use their own internal compass to guide their children and create their own visions and expectations for their children's future. Learning to ignore or counteract negative stereotypes and attitudes is part of this process.

**The Fishers:** Parents working together to build family unity and protect their children while allowing them to take healthy risks

D. K. and Erica were anticipating the birth of their first child with some anxiety. D. K. felt well prepared to be a parent, but Erica, although eager to begin a family, didn't feel as well equipped to be a mother. When Erica was six months pregnant with their first child, Dan, she and D. K. went for their prenatal doctor visit. After the examination, the nurse told them to wait to meet with the doctor. Because there were some irregularities on the sonogram, he referred them to a specialist, who diagnosed osteogenesis imperfecta (OI) in their unborn baby. They were not prepared for this news.

D. K. remembers seeing the pictures of Dan in utero. "I was shocked because I had been led to believe that all was fine. We had gone through all the checks and balances of pregnancy. My immediate thought was, How do we deal with it? We had no pity party. We didn't allow ourselves." He knew that OI was an uncommon disease that could make life complicated, so he started looking for treatments and cures; he wanted information. For Erica it was a "psychological adjustment."

When Dan was born, he had twelve broken bones. There was a sign on Dan's bassinet at the hospital: DO NOT TOUCH THIS BABY. D. K. and Erica carried Dan on a pillow for a year. Grandmother Ann, D. K.'s mother, was fearful: "How are we going to be able to do this?"

Other parents of kids with OI coached D. K. and Erica on how to explain Dan's fractures to medical personnel unfamiliar with OI. This was important in order to avoid suspicion of child abuse when taking Dan in for frequent broken bones. Because many doctors have no experience with this uncommon condition, D. K. and Erica have had to become very knowledgeable about OI. They have had to instruct doctors, especially in small-town hospitals, exactly how to treat their son. To help in medical emergencies, D. K. made and carries laminated cards with information about his son's diagnosis and treatment.

Erica found that everything in her life changed when she became a mother of a child who has a physical disability. "Nothing was normal." As a baby, Dan was so fragile that they were always on guard, especially around others who might be clumsy or not understand the risks, such as teenagers. They were afraid to use babysitters because of these risks; as a result, they had little couple relaxation time.

D. K. became the sole breadwinner when Erica gave up her profession to be a stay-at-home mother. As they gradually adapted to Dan's frequent bone breaks, their family life took on a routine, and they soon felt ready to have another child. Hank was born about a year later, and several years after that, they had daughter Sophie.

"Dan's brother and sister have been phenomenal. They are fabulous with their older brother." D. K. says that he and Erica have nurtured a sense of responsibility for others among the siblings. Hank and Sophie never let Dan feel he is imposing when he asks for anything. D. K. says that Dan is never a burden as "he has that no-quit attitude."

But Erica says it can sometimes be rough on Hank and Sophie. "Dan gets all the attention and Hank none. Then when there is a bone break I attend to Dan, and Hank has more responsibilities." Erica "coaches" D. K. in giving equal attention to each child. "She says, 'You're showing partiality to Dan'—and the other children have told me to be conscious of this," says D. K. He tries to talk with everyone at the dinner table and to participate in each child's activities. Grandmother Ann says that people pay attention to Dan while his siblings stand by quietly, deferring to their older brother. But that bothers Dan, so he speaks up for his siblings, reminding people who are talking to him that "I have a brother and a sister."

Erica says that she and D. K. help each other deal with Dan's multiple fractures, which come in waves. "We don't allow ourselves to get down. Having a strong spouse who doesn't wilt is a bonus," admits D. K. Erica appreciates that her husband is so even-keeled, keeping things light and happy. She also believes that she is a stronger person because of parenting three children, one who has a disability; sometimes she amazes herself. "Last summer Dan had two broken femurs. I slept on the floor with him. Then he broke his clavicle. People don't believe what I go through." D. K. says that he and Erica are "strong spouses for each other. No matter how painful, never did we show panic or fear. No matter how bad it is, we have it under control."

Erica and D. K. work together to keep the kids' spirits up when Dan has a broken bone. At those times, the family's schedule is often disrupted, and the children feel frustrated and sad when their plans have to be postponed or canceled. To lift the children's spirits, Erica always has special "stuff"—such as puzzles, DVDs, and books—ready for them to enjoy while she is busy attending to Dan.

All three children are good students and have varied interests. Dan, 14, is the family entertainer: "I love to make them smile." Dan also helps the family by using the Swiffer, making his bed, cleaning his room, and tutoring his younger sister. He likes making videos and is a good speaker, debater, and actor.

Hank, 12, says his role is to "help out" by vacuuming, raking the lawn, and helping Dan move around. Sometimes he carries Dan to another part of the room to play with the Xbox. He is close to Dan. He remembers getting upset once when Dan broke a bone; "I cried." Besides making straight As, he plays percussion in the school band and is on several sports teams, one of which is coached by Erica.

Sophie, at 9, says that she is "the one in my family with energy because I'm the littlest. Sleep is totally boring." She swims in the family pool with Dan because she feels that it makes him happy. Like Hank, she also plays on sports teams that Erica coaches or assists with. While Dan tutors her, Sophie likes to open doors for Dan and get him his glasses. Since she doesn't save her money, he uses his money to buy her candy. "His OI doesn't interfere with life. I feel completely good about it because everyone likes him."

The family swims and boats together. They installed an Endless Pool in their basement, forgoing other luxuries. In the summer they travel to their cabin, where they go boating on a lake. They "bubble jump" off the back of the boat. To protect his body against breaks, Dan keeps his limbs together when he jumps into the wake. Grandmother Ann says that Dan is allowed to take a kayak out alone at twilight to fish. "I am proud that his parents allow this."

Erica says that staying fit gives her the stamina to deal with emergencies as they arise. She swims half an hour each day to help maintain strength, and she enjoys running while listening to music. She finds social outlets coaching Hank's and Sophie's basketball and baseball teams and gets support from occasional meetings with friends. "Do for *you* once in a while," she advises. "It's the only way to keep it together."

The Fishers are an open, communicative, and active family. They believe in working for those causes they think are important. Erica and D. K. have been vocal advocates for OI since Dan was born, and their whole family is committed to raising funds for research on OI. D. K. feels strongly that "families have to be proactive about fund-raising in the race to find cures for disabilities." He is reaching out to big companies now, raising awareness of their social responsibility to contribute funds for disability research.

Grandmother Ann contributes to the cause by making baskets of donated goods to raise money for OI. "It keeps me busy. People have been donating to OI through me since Dan was born." She advises other grandparents to help as much as they can and to connect with and learn from others who are going through the same thing. She plays an important role in encouraging her son's family to *be* a family, and helping them to be a supportive one.

# 4

# Brothers and Sisters

## Siblings Sharing Family Life with Physical Disability in the Mix

"We're all people. We just have different things in common. That's good because otherwise we'd all be the same."

—ISABEL, THIRD OF FOUR SIBS

"We have a good relationship, but we fight like all sisters."

—ELIZA, OLDEST OF FOUR SISTERS

Relationships between brothers and sisters are the most enduring of all family ties, often lasting a lifetime, and yet they've gotten the "short end of the stick" when it comes to research on families. Sibling connections remain somewhat mysterious; no one really knows what's "normal" in *any* sibling alliance. So it's hard to say whether sibling relationships in a family that includes a child who has a physical disability are different from or more "difficult" than those in any other family.

Some research studies have explored experiences of able-bodied siblings who have a brother or sister who has a disability, but very few have included the perspective of the sibling who *has* the disability. Instead of trying to understand the relationship *between* the siblings, most studies focus on how the able-bodied sibling is affected emotionally and socially *by* the brother or sister who has a disability. In the past, most people, including social scientists, assumed that able-bodied children would suffer negative effects as a result of having a sibling who has a physical disability—so that's what they looked for. But this is not the case. In reality, studies that compare children whose sibling has a disability with those who have only able-bodied siblings show that there are no differences in their psychological or social adjustment.

This doesn't mean that relationships between able-bodied siblings and those who have disabilities are all smooth sailing or without challenges. Siblings have mixed feelings about *all* their brothers and sisters. When a family includes a child who has a physical disability, all the siblings have a chance to develop patience, compassion for others, and good social skills, but they may—or may not!—also experience more worry, stress, jealousy, or conflict. It all depends on the circumstances of the family, the way parents handle the situation, and the personalities of each individual child.

This chapter explores how you can set the stage for good sibling relationships among your children by modeling positive attitudes, paying equal attention to each child, including all the sibs in family activities, and assigning age- and ability-appropriate responsibilities to each child. This is followed by a look at sibling relationships from the point of view of both able-bodied sibs and those who have disabilities—how siblings help and share with each other, how they cope with problems, and how they find support.

## Parents Set the Stage

Parents' attitudes toward disability have a major influence on the quality of relationships between siblings in families that include able-bodied kids and those who have disabilities. Inclusive parents have a positive attitude toward each of their children and want *all* of them to enjoy the benefits of sibling camaraderie by taking part in family activities. They expect their child who has a disability to share in responsibilities and achieve individual goals, just like his siblings. When parents help their child who has a disability fully participate in his sibling role, his able-bodied siblings are likely to be better adjusted, too.

One way to set the stage for good sibling relationships in your family is by making a conscious effort to give equal attention, affection, and quality time to each of your children, despite extra requirements that your child who has a physical disability may have. Able-bodied siblings may grumble, but deep down they understand that the physical disability of their brother or sister sometimes demands more parental time or energy. They are usually aware and appreciative of their parents' efforts to balance the time they give to each child—even when the results are not perfect. Michelle, whose older sister Eliza (who has CP) is now away at college, was often unhappy about the energy drain on her parents because of Eliza's needs. Yet she valued her parents' emotional involvement with all the sisters, as well as the fact that, for the most part, they "didn't overlook any of our needs, or problems in our lives; they supported our activities." Her younger sister Alice agrees that all the girls "get equal attention. No one person is favored."

Kids who have a disability benefit when their parents include them in the day-to-day life of the family—both routine and fun activities. When you create opportunities for shared sibling experiences, you encourage "bonding" between sibs that leads to closer and more caring relationships. One way to do this is to identify a sport or activity that all children can enjoy together. The Fishers, for example, made swimming a focal point for family fun and exercise, because all their children enjoyed the family pool and it was safe for their son Dan, who has OI. In the Jones family, everyone likes miniature golf, and it's an activity in which all the children are able to participate. They also create a family vegetable garden, a fun family project, where they can spend time together and produce something that everyone shares and enjoys. They prepare the garden plot in the spring and plant their jointly agreed-upon crops; in the summer, they take turns watering and weeding. Angie, who uses a wheelchair, sits on the ground to work in the dirt alongside her older brothers and sisters.

When parents assign similar, if not identical, responsibilities to each child in the family and enforce the same standards of ethics and social behavior for each of them, they set up an inclusive team. Eliza, whose *physical* needs took more parental attention than those of her sibs, appre-

> **T** To make gardening more accessible, build elevated containers for plants that are at wheelchair height. This creates an "equal opportunity" garden: the whole family can use this raised garden to share in planting, weeding, and playing in the soil!

ciates that when it comes to other areas of her development, "I've had the same guidelines as my sisters; there is no special treatment." Her parents expect her to reach the same goals for academic achievement and uphold the same moral codes as her sisters—and eventually to become a socially and emotionally independent adult, in spite of her physical limitations.

Even with the best of intentions, it's not a good idea to let your child who has a physical disability avoid responsibilities, or to lavish excessive attention on him. In fact, as Fred points out, "doting on the one who has a disability" is not good for *any* of the children. "The one who has the disability doesn't want it, and it causes dependency by the child who has the disability and resentment in the others." This can create a "spoiled" child, whose "special" treatment gets in the way of her ability to develop competence and independence. If your child who has a disability is pampered, protected, and allowed to dominate your attentions, she is more likely to become bossy and demanding—traits not leading to good sibling relationships! On the other hand, she may feel guilty about her siblings' unfair load of responsibilities or their relative neglect by parents and unjustly blame herself for being a "burden." Fred's parents were careful *not* to overindulge or baby his sister who had a physical disability. Because Fred's sister "pitched in to help with the household chores, there was no extra burden on the other kids," and sibling relationships were good.

When you expect your child who has a disability to take on chores and responsibilities equivalent (in proportion to her physical abilities) to those of her able-bodied sibs, your children are less likely to have conflicts or jealousies related to special treatment of the child who has a disability. Priscilla Brandon, whose son has spina bifida, embraces the philosophy of evenhanded parenting. "Don't make the child with the disability the center," she says. "All children need responsibilities and discipline—no one person has entitlements." Priscilla's daughter Jean, who is able-bodied, appreciates her parents' policy of "treating all children evenly and not sheltering either child." She and her brother who has spina bifida were each expected to excel in school, to keep their rooms clean, and to follow family standards for minding their manners and keeping their tempers in check. The Brandons' expectations of each child are coupled with their willingness to give each child the support needed to achieve his or her goals. For Jason this included advocating for accessibility and personal care attendants at his college, while for Jean it meant "pushing me in my chosen path"—to become an actress—and "coming to all my performances." Jean reports a loving relationship with Jason and says that there is little jealousy between them.

The Fishers assign chores to each of their children, based on their abilities. Fourteen-year-old Dan, though physically limited by OI, is expected to sweep floors, make his bed, clean his room, and help his younger sister with her homework. His 12-year-old brother, Hank, who is able-bodied, does more strenuous chores, like raking leaves and vacuuming, while 9-year-old Sophie sets the dinner table and loads the dishwasher. These siblings each describe their relationships as close and loving. Says Dan, "We get along really well; we do well together. Most other siblings aren't as close as we are." Hank enjoys "a lot of laughs" in his relationship with Dan and Sophie, as well as feeling empathy for Dan's struggle. "When Dan broke a bone, I cried. My brother and I are close." Sophie looks up to and feels protected by both of her older brothers. She can count on Dan, the oldest, for special treats. "He buys me candy and we play Xbox together."

Of course, expectations for the child who has a disability have to be realistic. Some families assume that fair treatment means exactly the same treatment for all sibs, and they hold the unrealistic expectation that the child who has a disability must match his siblings' contributions in *every* way. If the child is not able to live up to those expectations, she may blame herself for being a "failure." It is useful for parents to think about giving each child responsibilities that match his or her age and abilities, rather than assigning *identical* responsibilities to every child. Margo has her children change the sheets on their beds on the weekends. Her 12-year-old daughter who uses crutches struggles with this, so Margo had all the siblings work out a swap that they thought was fair—while her sibs changed their sister's bed for her, the 12-year-old sister put pillowcases on all of their pillows and dusted the bedrooms.

When parents raise their children to expect that they will be asked for help at appropriate times, their children, including the child who has the physical disability, can be counted on to help one another when needed. If children regularly help their parents or sibs as part of their age-appropriate role in the family, and if they are rewarded with love and attention, they may become more compassionate and caring adults and learn the value of being responsible for another person.

The trick for parents is identifying chores that their children who have disabilities can do to help siblings and the family. Some parents expect an older sibling who has a physical disability to help with the care or supervision of their able-bodied younger sibs. Chores such as helping younger sibs with homework or babysitting are common. When siblings share in the care of their brothers or sisters, it gives their parents more free time and energy to spend on fun and interesting activities and interactions with *all* the children.

Other things that parents have found helpful in setting the stage for good sibling relationships include encouraging open communication and sharing among family members, making sure that all siblings have ample opportunities for recreation and fun, and using humor to defuse conflicts and bring a healthy perspective to the family.

But parents are only a part of the story. No matter how evenhanded parents are, siblings will still fight with one another, be envious, and feel that another sib was given special attention or treatment that they were not. And in some families where there is not enough attention or support for the children, siblings will band together and become exceptionally close.

Every child's relationship to his parents will be different. Parents gain experience and wisdom as they have more children, mature as individuals, and experience changes in their economic, marital, or other life circumstances. Sometimes family size plays a role; in larger families, the emotional impact of one child who has a disability may be more easily "absorbed" and have less influence on sibling relationships. Finally, each child comes with his own "hard-wired" temperament that interacts in unique ways with parents' and siblings' personalities and relationship styles.

As anyone who has a brother or sister knows, relationships between them have a life of their own, separate from each sib's relationship with their parents. They can love each other to pieces; fight like cats and dogs; share experiences, dreams, and secrets; envy and resent each other; and help, support, and protect one another. In spite—or because—of these early experiences of companionship and conflict, brothers and sisters grow into mature and competent adults.

## Jealousy, Guilt, and Sibling Rivalry

The O'Brien family includes Eliza, who has CP, and her three younger sisters. Their parents tried hard to find recreational activities that *everyone* in the family could do together. But this meant that the younger girls had to give up some activities they were interested in, since Eliza was physically unable to do them. They felt that this wasn't fair, even though they knew their parents were trying hard to do the right thing. Sister Alice says that because Eliza's been "confined to her room through so many surgeries," her parents put a TV in her room, while none of the other girls have one. The girls understand the rationale, but they still feel jealous. Eliza is very close to her mother, and Alice worries that mom's intense involvement with Eliza might take away from her relationships with the other sisters. But the girls love Eliza, they want to protect her, and they feel guilty about being able to enjoy so much that Eliza cannot.

Sam, who had polio as a child, recalls that his brothers were jealous of his relationship with their father, while he was envious of the attention they got from their mother (who had rejected Sam because of his disability). But despite vying for parental attention, Sam and his brothers were close; his middle brother in particular was always "nice to me; he was supportive and cheered me up."

Ashley, the youngest of three siblings, was 17 at the time of her injury. Her siblings also "competed" for their mother's attention. Marie recalls that her middle child was jealous because Ashley "consumed my time and energy; she needed me." After the accident, Ashley's parents stopped taking the family on beach vacations because Ashley's disability made it difficult for her to get to the beach. When Ashley's able-bodied sibs had to give up an enjoyable experience, they felt more resentment, and Ashley felt guilty for getting in the way of their enjoyment. Yet when Ashley was a young adult engaged to be married, and her family went to Disney World without her, she still felt "jealous that they could go" and she couldn't. Ashley notes that she and her sibs did not talk openly about these difficult feelings—and that this "made things worse for my family."

## Talking Things Through

Communication between siblings is vital for creating close relationships, learning to deal with conflicts, and having fun. Early on, talking allows children to play games, to "make believe," and to develop friendships. In the preteen and teen years, kids love to talk about relationships— siblings enjoy discussing the ways that each one relates to their parents or close friends and dissecting their parents' relationship to each other. Siblings aren't just being nosey. When they "gossip" about relationships, they are actually coping with complex feelings, understanding relationship conflicts, and thinking about solutions. And they are reinforcing a sense of connection to their family.

When a child's ability to participate in sports or other physical activities is limited by a disability or injury, talking can become even more important to forging connections and sharing experiences with their siblings. Alice finds that of her three sisters, she talks the most with Eliza. They share many interests, including history, TV shows, and spectator sports, and Alice says that Eliza "is the calmest in the family, easy to talk with." Eliza and Michelle weren't always able to talk freely, but since Eliza went away to college, she can "talk about more things with Michelle, perhaps because we don't compete for attention at home anymore." With her youngest sister, Sammi, Eliza finds that "I'm able to help her—she talks to me." When Sammi struggles with schoolwork, Eliza says, "I'm more understanding and patient. I'm good at relating to people so maybe I'm the sounding board."

## Sharing Experiences

In most families, some activities are shared by all the siblings, while others are one-on-one between a child and a parent. Generally, as children get older, more activities are shared with friends outside the family. A disability can lead to increased social exposure for a child—whether because of more time spent in academic or rehabilitation settings, being involved in disability or advocacy groups, or just responding to the curiosity of people encountering a young person in a wheelchair or on crutches. As Eliza says, "I've met lots of different people through my disability." But having a disability can also limit opportunities to create close friendships, especially if it causes frequent medical problems, hospitalizations, or prolonged periods of recovery. Sibling friendships are especially important in these situations.

Dan, who has OI, has frequent bone breaks and often needs to stay home for several weeks to recover. Although Dan is popular at school, his able-bodied brother Hank says that Dan "doesn't have lots of friends outside of school, so I hang out with him. My brother and I are close. We substitute computer games for playing ball together." When Dan is well, he and Hank go on "boys only" fishing trips with their dad. When the family goes trail riding, Dan joins in with his siblings, riding in a cart pulled by Hank's bicycle.

Sometimes the sib who has a disability enjoys "going along for the ride" even if he can't participate in the chosen activity. Sam enjoyed watching his brothers go sledding, even though he couldn't sled because of having polio. "I admired my brothers; they brought excitement to my life."

Age differences between brothers and sisters can influence the activities they do together. Zoey, a 16-year-old, has a 4-year-old sister who has OI and says, "She loves me to fix her hair and to play dolls with her." At 9, Isabel rewards her little sister by playing video games with her. "I let her play with them when she does something good." Zoey, Isabel, and their brother Joseph enjoy watching movies together and cooperate in cleaning their rooms.

A family's resources also play a role in the types of activities that siblings share. Janet's mother, a university professor, was able to travel extensively during sabbaticals from teaching, bringing the children along. "We went to Scotland when I was 7 and in a wheelchair," Janet recalls. She shared many good times with her brother during trips to Holland and France, where they visited cultural sites and museums, went on tours of the cities, and ate wonderful meals.

> "Siblings should treat the person who has a disability like the others. Go places where people who have disabilities can go; don't go separately."
> —Alice

For Cora, whose dad was a factory foreman, quality time with her sibs was simpler, but just as special—Sunday picnics in the park with the whole family and spring vacations at her grandparents' house near the beach. Cora's big brother Toby would push her in a "sand chair"—a wheelchair fitted with oversize tires—so she could get down near the water. Cora, Toby, and little brother Al spent hours looking for shells and sand dollars, and when it was time to swim, Cora's grandfather would come down and carry her into the water with the other kids.

## Helping Each Other

When one child has a physical disability, some amount of help from able-bodied siblings is normal and may be necessary to the smooth functioning of the family. In many families, the degree of help is similar to what happens in any family, where older siblings help younger ones, or sibs work together to complete projects or chores. In others, able-bodied siblings need to go the "extra mile" for their sibling who has a disability. In families where mutual help and support are a family norm, children usually want to help; in these families, the sibling who has a disability, depending on her age and abilities, also helps her able-bodied sibs. Helping a sibling is a source of pride and enjoyment, though in some situations the need to help can cause resentment. Most sibs experience both pros and cons in helping their brothers or sisters.

Erik's parents divorced when he was very young. After living with his dad for a year, he moved in permanently with his mother, Jesse. He was 8 years old when Jesse and her partner, Lynn, adopted a daughter who had multiple disabilities; two more daughters who had disabilities were added to the family over the next few years. Erik was old enough to help out and to appreciate the pressing care needs of his sisters. "I've never felt my needs diminished by my little sisters. Their needs may be life and death. How would I feel if I put my needs first, and something happened to them?" Of course, there were times, when things were particularly hectic, that Erik felt "like a servant" and longed to be "left alone." But since he was so young when his family went through radical changes (his parents divorced, his mother moved in with her partner, and three girls who had disabilities joined the family), Erik "expects chaos in life."

In retrospect, Erik recognizes that he had a tendency to do too much; he had to learn "when my help could be a hindrance and I needed to back off." Erik also knows that his personality makes it easy for people to lean on him, sometimes too much. "I'd sometimes like to feel less appreciated. People think I have the right answer. I listen and don't judge; I don't make waves. I'm the nice guy."

Now a young man, Erik still feels a strong sense of family unity that incorporates his sisters' needs. "Our norms are different. There are challenges we face as a group—we adapt things to fit our life." But he also enjoys an independent social life, has a full-time job, and is working on his first novel. Although he was very involved in the care of his sisters, Erik doesn't feel that his family held him back; in fact, he says that they helped him grow "by showing me how life is, and guiding me into the real world."

For Erik, taking care of his sisters was a mixed bag, but on the whole it was a positive experience. At times he felt that too much help was expected of him, and he had difficulty asserting his own needs, which seemed insignificant next to his sisters' life-and-death medical issues. On the other hand, Erik was proud of his ability to adapt to change and to do his part for the good of the family. He developed greater empathy, flexibility, and tolerance that served him well as he became an adult.

Michelle sometimes felt frustrated or resentful as a result of her family's expectation that she help Eliza, especially when she felt she had to put her sister's needs ahead of her own. "Eliza went to physical therapy camps in the summer," she says, "so we had to spend summers in the car taking her there."

For Paige, resentment and anger about taking care of her sister were caused by her parents' inability to create a safe environment for their children and her having to take on more responsibilities than any child should. Her siblings' survival depended on Paige becoming a "step-in mother," and she felt overwhelmed by having to care for them. Children put in this position miss the chance to have fun with their siblings and feel robbed of their childhoods; they can feel, as Paige did, like "the little maid." Family situations like Paige's can cause feelings of deprivation, jealousy, and resentment; create emotional distance between siblings; and make it difficult to form friendships outside the family.

The oldest of three siblings, Paige is now a young woman. She recalls her family as "chaotic, irrational, non-nurturing, and unstable"; she "grew up quickly without much of a childhood." Paige's younger sister had spina bifida, and her baby brother had autism and severe intellectual disability. Her father left the family when she was little, then moved back in, but was abusive to Paige's mother and neglectful of the children. Paige became the "mother figure" for her siblings. She helped take care of them and did many household chores. When she was younger, she felt very close to her siblings, but as they got older, "the relationship soured." Paige resented being the child who always had to "take up the slack," because her parents were inadequate and had low expectations of her sister. "I had animosity, not toward my sister, just about the situation."

Looking back, Paige wishes that her parents had encouraged her sister to take more risks and responsibilities, so she could have become more confident. And she wishes they could have understood her perspective as the able-bodied child. On the positive side, Paige found that as a result of caring for her siblings, she was more prepared to be a mother herself. She makes a conscious effort to raise her own children differently than she was raised, giving them emotional support and attention, respecting their views and feelings, and having regular "family time."

For Zoey, an able-bodied 16-year-old and the oldest of four siblings, helping her youngest sibling, who has OI, has been primarily a positive experience, partly because she shares the job with two other able-bodied sibs. Their parents recently divorced, and their mother has to work long hours. Zoey is in charge when their mother is out. "I'm the oldest. I watch everyone while Mom's at work. I hold down the fort." While this involves some special care for her sister who has OI, Zoey doesn't resent having this responsibility. "If Mom needs me one Friday night, she is lenient on another night"; Zoey is not expected to sacrifice her social life in order to babysit her siblings. Additionally, her mother appreciates Zoey's help and "lets me know I'm a good kid. I don't go un-thanked."

Her 13-year-old brother, Joseph, the only son and self-proclaimed "man of the house," also cares for his two younger sisters, "babysitting and playing board games" with them. When his youngest sister was born with OI, Joseph says he "got more chores, but I didn't mind. Sometimes I was out playing and then I'd have to come inside to watch my baby sister." On the other hand, Joseph thought, "it was cool to have a new member of the family. She looked up to me."

Sister Isabel, age 9, waxes philosophical in discussing their baby sister's disability. "You can't pick everything you want in your life," she says. She knows that "the job of keeping her safe is painful and stressful for everyone in the family." But, like Joseph, she acknowledges that being an older sib who pitches in to help the family run smoothly makes her feel important and valued. "Every day I tell myself to do some extra chore. Sometimes I do extra things to help Mom. I like the feeling of doing something good."

In the Fisher family, younger sister Sophie helps Dan, who has OI, by "opening doors for him and getting his glasses," and younger brother Hank helps move him about, sometimes carrying him. Dan, on the other hand, has the job of helping his younger siblings with their homework. Dan does not see himself as a "burden," nor do his siblings; they consider the different types of helping they do to be part of the normal give and take in their particular family.

In most families, the child who has a physical disability is able to help the able-bodied siblings in various ways, as well as accepting their help when needed. This may be especially true if the sib who has a disability is older than the other children. Janet, who has spina bifida and uses a wheelchair, had a younger brother and stepsister. Although "it was a challenge for me to care for them physically," one of Janet's responsibilities in the family was to help with her little stepsister. Janet appreciated the fact that caring went both ways between her and her siblings. "When kids made fun of me, my brother stood up for me"; as they have grown older, Janet feels that her good relationship with her siblings has become even closer. Janet advises families to encourage able-bodied siblings to help care for their sib who has a disability, but she believes it's equally important for the sib who has a disability to help care for a younger one, if possible. Her experiences of getting help and giving help in her family have made her "a more caring person."

Sometimes the sibling who has a disability becomes responsible for brothers and sisters when parents are emotionally absent, neglectful, or abusive. Even in these situations, the sibling who has a disability, just like an able-bodied sib, can benefit from the chance to be a giver, as well as a receiver, of help.

Emma recalls that her spina bifida was "the straw that broke the camel's back" for her emotionally unstable mother. Her parents fought frequently and were unable to cooperate in her care. They separated, but during a brief period of reconciliation, her mother became pregnant with Emma's brother; he was born when Emma was 8. When her brother was 2 years old, her father left the family for good. Emma's mother was unable to manage the load of work, home, and child care responsibilities; they ate carryout food every night, and Emma's mom would often forget to buy food or to give them lunch money for school. When her mother started dating again, she left the children home alone. So Emma became the protector and substitute mom for her little brother. She took loans from friends to buy him food, and she made sure he was clean and properly dressed for school. She watched over him when her mother was gone and gave him as much emotional support as she could.

Eventually, her mother's boyfriend moved in with them, but he soon became verbally abusive, and the children felt unsafe around him. Emma and her brother went to live with her father at that point. Because he lived in a rough neighborhood, where waiting for the school bus could be unsafe, Emma had to continue protecting both her brother and herself from harm.

Helping her little brother had some benefits—her brother never thought her disability lessened Emma's competence, and caring for her brother helped shape her career choice. Now a mother herself and a school teacher, Emma used her course work in human development to help her design a plan for being a good parent. She is a nurturing mom who tries to be caring and protective without "micromanaging."

Though Emma has a physical disability and Paige is able-bodied, they each played extraordinary roles in caring for a younger sibling, primarily as the result of parental neglect. Like Paige, Emma views her childhood experiences as a model for what *not* to do. "I do nothing like my parents," she says. "My memories guide me day to day, correcting my childhood."

Emma and Paige are among the "invulnerables," children who become resilient and capable adults in spite of neglect or abuse in childhood. In other families where parents are struggling with poverty, divorce, substance abuse, or mental illness, children may experience more difficulty coping with ups and downs in their sibling relationships. Felicity, for example, grew up with alcoholic parents, and her mother was abusive. At age 19, she had a spinal cord injury, and in the absence of any guidance or support from parents, her siblings reacted badly. She recalls that her "youngest sister didn't visit her much" while she was in the rehabilitation hospital, and when she did, "she would complain and whine" about her own problems, unable to offer emotional support to Felicity. Her middle sister "took my injury hard and got into drugs." These sibs had no support to cope with Felicity's injury or to handle life's challenges.

## "Cope-ability" for Sibs

When children who have physical disabilities and their able-bodied sibs are raised by caring and capable parents, *all* can learn to cope with problems, thrive, and become productive adults. In addition to good parenting, some other factors that improve the "cope-ability" of siblings are good communication, positive belief systems, the ability to redefine themselves, and support from peers.

## Communication

Communication is a cornerstone of resilient families. Siblings who can communicate more openly and directly about their thoughts and feelings are generally better able to cope and solve problems. Sharing feelings with each other, their parents, or friends helps sibs deal with highs and lows of daily life.

Isabel likes "to keep relationships strong in the family, to be a good family," and she is a big fan of communication as a means to this end. But in a busy family with four sibs, Isabel sometimes has to struggle to be heard. "I get upset when people cut me off when I am talking. That happens a lot." Isabel copes by communicating with her mother, even if no one else is listening. This helps her get relief from frustrating situations and figure out how to solve problems in her relationships with her siblings or others in her life. "Sometimes I get so aggravated that things explode in my mind. I don't like holding it in, it's not a way to settle things. I say what's bothering me. I talk with Mom and I let it out. Then it's not all up in my mind." Eliza agrees that sharing feelings is a good way to cope. "Don't bottle up feelings and then explode; communicate," she says. While Isabel finds solace in talking to Mom, her sister Zoey turns to friends and her church community. "I go to Mass with my two best friends. We talk about our problems and it's better than coping alone."

Interestingly, siblings don't always communicate directly about the disability itself. In a study of over forty siblings of children who have a physical disability, almost half said they didn't talk about the disability at all—either because they were uncomfortable bringing up the subject or because the child who had the disability preferred not to discuss it. In some families, it may not be needed or important to discuss the disability, or disability may be overshadowed by other pressing problems. Emma recalls that she and her brother "never had a conversation about my disability. During his formative years too many things were going on: our parents split up, we lived with our mother's boyfriend, and I was my brother's babysitter much of the time." Sometimes the impact of a sibling's disability is communicated in roundabout ways; Janet remembers that although they did not openly discuss her disability, "my brother wrote a story about me and my disability for his college application essay."

## Spirituality

Spirituality is one way of coping that is important to many children, as it is to adults. Praying, "talking" to God, and practicing religious rituals can give children a feeling of comfort and security. Zoey, whose youngest sib has OI, describes herself as "the religious one" in her family. "I do a church retreat where the teen group sleeps in the church on the weekend. You have to be sponsored, and then you belong." Zoey's religious affiliation is both an expression of faith and a way to get support from and fit in with her peers, so important to teenagers.

Eliza's faith has helped her deal with disappointments in life, some related to having CP. "When I got mad because life hadn't worked out the way I wanted, I thought of the good things that happened." Eliza's appreciation of the good things in her life is linked with her belief that "someone up there is watching." Eliza goes to church almost every Sunday and belongs to a Catholic club at her college. When she needs help or support, she "says a Hail Mary."

Sam found religion in college. He remembers the night he was "called," sitting in the balcony of a church. He volunteered to be saved and decided to become a minister. After years of exposure to prejudice and social isolation because of his disability, Sam experienced "being accepted and belonging" through religion; it made him feel "at home in the universe" for the first time.

Darlene was raised Catholic but rejected the formal teachings of the church when she was about 12 years old. Darlene found her own brand of spirituality, combining various religious traditions. "I have a touch of Catholicism, a touch of Buddhism, a little Islam. I'm spiritual in my own way. It's made me feel better about helping my sister Wanda, who has quadriplegia. I believe in karma; I do good deeds and hope they will come back to me."

Not all children (or their families) believe in a higher power. But many kids find solace in their connection to the natural world or strength in identifying as a "citizen of the universe," experiences that have a spiritual quality. Nikki, a 10-year-old whose sister Jodi lost both legs in a car accident, says that when she's having a bad day, she goes for a walk in the woods near her house and listens to the birds. "There's a special spot where I sit on a big rock and see rays of light coming in through the trees, and I just feel like I'm part of something bigger than me. I kind of forget to be sad about Jodi and think about how beautiful and amazing the world is." Nikki's brother Bob likes to camp out in the summers, and he took Nikki and Jodi on an overnight trip at an accessible campground he had found. Bob says, "It was awesome. You realize you're all spinning around in space with the stars and planets. It's a great feeling!"

Eli, a teen who walks with crutches as a result of CP, got involved with a nonprofit that provides health care for children in Africa and helps their mothers start small businesses. He started out as a local fund-raiser and eventually traveled to Africa to spend a summer volunteering in a small village. Eli's perspective on his place in the world was totally changed. "I'm not just a 'little guy' dealing with everyday hassles—I'm helping families on another continent, and I'm seeing great results firsthand. It makes me feel stronger; people respect me for what I do and they don't care if I can't walk perfectly. I'm not into religion at all, but I think my life will turn out better because I'm connected to so many people in a good way."

## Reframing Who You Are

As we have seen, children who have disabilities and their able-bodied siblings redefine what is "normal" for themselves and their family. They often reframe the disability experience to keep it from "spreading," that is, to make sure the disability—or having a sib who has a disability—won't become the central fact of their personal identity. Frequently, siblings attribute some positive character traits to the positive effects of disability.

Eliza says she knows her "disability is a big deal, but I don't make it a big deal. I always say I may not like being in a wheelchair but if I weren't I would be a different person. I like being me. Disability is just a part of me."

Arthur and his twin brother share a congenital muscle disorder causing weakness and poor coordination. The twins required special medical care and intensive physical therapy in early childhood; his mother gave them little prizes when they did their physical therapy exercises, and Arthur recalls that he never thought about it as being "a drag." As an adult,

Arthur has some weakness that limits his physical abilities, but he defines himself by what he can do and what he enjoys—intellectual pursuits, science, playing the cello, cycling, playing with his dog, and being a father to his children. Having an identical twin who shared his disability made him feel less alone and different; he always "fit in" with his twin. In addition, Arthur had good relationships with his two older brothers and didn't see himself as "a problem" because of his disability. While not the defining force in his life, his disability is a factor in his "forward-looking" approach. "I've developed into a can-do person in every aspect of my life; I don't throw in the towel."

The realization that disability does not define you as a person is important for both able-bodied siblings and those who have disabilities. Seeing yourself as a person who is quiet, interested in sharks, a Yankees fan, a fly fisher, a medium student, and, oh yes, someone who uses a wheelchair helps you incorporate disability into your life without having it take over. You don't deny it, but you don't let it crowd out all the good and interesting things in your life.

As Michelle points out, able-bodied siblings also have weaknesses, challenges, and "special" needs. The experience of having a sib who has a disability can help able-bodied children learn to be more tolerant of their own imperfections or problems and to put them in perspective—focusing more on their strengths and abilities. One expression of their "cope-ability" is siblings' choice of the "lens" that lets them view the person first and then the disability—and not necessarily to identify it as a flaw, but just a part of the bigger picture.

### Making Friends with People Who "Get It"

Finding a friend who has a disability or a friend whose sibling has a disability can be difficult, and many children feel somewhat alone with their family's experience of disability. But as Zoey reports, it's easier to find friends who have *someone* who has a disability in their family, even if it's not a sibling. Zoey's kinship with these friends helps validate her ideas about disability, which are at odds with the stereotypes of most of her peers. "I have a different view of people who have a disability. I can share this with people at school who have family members who have disabilities. We have that connection." Friendships with peers who share their disability experience help children feel understood and give them a sense of belonging.

### Support Groups for Siblings

Informal support from friends is especially valuable for siblings, since there are few formal support groups available for them. One notable exception, the "Sibshop" program, aims to fill that gap. Its developers note that, "for most parents, the thought of 'going it alone'—raising a child with special needs without the benefit of knowing another parent in a similar situation—would be unthinkable. Yet this routinely happens to brothers and sisters. It is not uncommon for siblings to be in their forties before they meet others who share their unique joys and concerns. Forty years is a long time to wait for validation."

Not all children need or want this type of group experience. Some get adequate support from their friends and family. Others feel uncomfortable in groups and may do better with individual counseling, if they need more support than friends and family can provide. But many children can benefit from peer support, particularly if their opportunity to find understanding friends is limited. If you think that your children would benefit, contact the Sibling Support Project (see Resources section of this book), which conducts Sibshops at locations around the country. Sibling (and parent) advocacy efforts could potentially help to develop more local support programs for siblings of kids who have disabilities. Interested siblings could approach disability organizations or local rehabilitation hospitals to start a support group in their community. Other places to hold informal support groups are schools, churches, and community centers.

## Growing Together

Siblings who have a disability frequently experience positive changes in their personality—such as greater sensitivity toward others, increased tolerance for diversity, more appreciation for their abilities, and striving to be better people. Arthur's physical disability spurred his "constant drive to be better . . . to rise above my physical limitations." Eliza's disability has made her more "appreciative . . . a more open person. I'm a lot more understanding." Ashley says that her experiences with disability "showed me that lots of people are better off or worse off than I am. It taught me to deal with things, how to cope." Felicity says, "I am blessed. I may not walk, but I can use my arms and move my legs." Coping with her disability, including the negative reactions of her siblings, has given Felicity a sense of competence and self-awareness. "We're the strong ones," she says. "We're a lot wiser than those walking around looking at us."

Children who have a brother or sister who has a physical disability experience similar kinds of personal growth. When asked about the positive effects of having a sibling who has a disability, they frequently mention increased tolerance for individual differences, greater empathy and compassion for others, and more appreciation of their health and abilities. Other character traits associated with being the sib of a person who has a disability are patience, kindness, insight into coping with challenges, dependability, and loyalty. Siblings who act as advocates can also develop greater assertiveness, self-confidence, and persistence.

"As a kid I used to play with a little girl who was mentally retarded and it was no big deal. She was one of us." —Michelle, whose older sister has a disability

Jean reports that her brother's disability has had an "impact on our view of the world," making her family more compassionate and concerned, not just about disability but about other social and environmental issues. "It's made our family more emotional about the world. We are disappointed about global warming and wars." Jean feels that her "brother made me a better person."

Charlie, Fred, and Sukey are three of five sibs; their sister had a childhood illness resulting in a physical disability. For them, the impact of having a sister who has a physical disability was woven into their experiences as part of a large, active, and supportive sibling group. Charlie, the third-born, says his interactions with his sister made him more compassionate, "made people respect me," and led to a feeling of solidarity, not just with his sister but with all people who have disabilities. "I am a more humane person; I have more human feelings for those who have less. I side with them."

"I don't fear disability; I don't look and judge a book by its cover." —Paige, whose two younger sibs have disabilities

Oldest brother Fred, who drove his sister to high school and got her wheelchair out of the car, also feels good about how his relationship with his sister affected him. "I was proud. I made things possible for her, and was happy. It made me a better person." Their youngest sister, Sukey, says, "I grew up during the JFK era—things were to be equal for everyone. I felt that people who had disabilities were part of that." Although she was much younger than her oldest sister, "I felt protective when I walked with her. We would hold pinkies. When kids stared, my sister would look down at me and say, 'It doesn't matter.' Now I go out of my way to acknowledge people who have disabilities."

As adults, Charlie, Fred, and Sukey place a high value on their sibling relationships. Like Jean's family, their worldview expanded, in part because of having a sister who has a physical disability. Fred notes, "The impact on our family was definitely positive. We are all more open-minded and understanding." And Sukey says, "I felt so lucky to have the family I do. My family enriched my life."

### The Brandons: A family devoted to faith, education, and unconditional love, inspired by Grandfather's example and bolstered by his support

D isability is normal to us, part of our daily routine. It's not a bad thing, you know," says Jean, a teen who doesn't view her brother's spina bifida (SB) as a problem. She reflects her family's attitude that Jason's disability is just a part of life.

Grandfather Frank is a vital member of the Brandon family, ready to lend a hand anytime. Frank and his wife were always supportive, stepping in to help whenever the family needed them. But when Frank's wife died several years ago, he admits, "I buried myself in the grandkids."

Frank became a regular part of the family's life. He helped Jason get ready for school each morning while parents Lee and Priscilla got ready for work (Lee owns a construction business, and Priscilla works for the school system), and then he drove Jean and Jason to and from school. Frank continues this routine with Jean, now that Jason is away at college. Although he has a long commute to the Brandon home, the time and effort are worth it to Frank; the love and respect he receives from his grandchildren give him great pleasure and have helped him adjust to life without his wife.

Priscilla's first pregnancy ended in a miscarriage of twins following a car accident. After that, she was cautious and watched her health carefully. She soon became pregnant again, but by the twenty-eighth week, she hadn't felt the baby move. Priscilla pleaded with her obstetrician to prescribe an ultrasound, but the doctor refused because it was not covered by insurance. But the doctor's face revealed concern, and when Lee said he would pay out of pocket, the doctor sent Priscilla for a scan.

At the hospital, medical staff gathered to observe the ultrasound. There was silence except when the technician asked, "What's this?" That night the doctor called to tell the Brandons their baby might have SB. It was the worst day of Lee's life; he felt frightened. He wanted to protect his wife and his unborn child, but there was nothing he could do. Priscilla also felt helpless. After that she had an ultrasound every two weeks to check on the baby's condition.

The Brandons were referred to the local Spina Bifida Association (SBA) chapter and invited to a barbeque to meet other families. They felt overwhelmed by the wide range of abilities of the children with SB and wondered where their child would fit along this spectrum.

They were also referred to a geneticist, who warned them that the baby might have brain damage. After leaving his office, Priscilla cried for forty-five minutes in the parking lot. When she dried her tears, she resolved to educate herself, delving into research on SB.

Priscilla contacted a surgeon, whom she describes as "so wonderful." He explained that hydrocephalus is treatable and that brain damage can often be prevented. "Wait until you have this beautiful baby. You're going to love him and play with him and cherish every moment you have with him. Leave his medical care to me." That put everything in perspective for Priscilla.

Two weeks before the due date, Priscilla delivered Jason by C-section. He seemed so fragile that Priscilla "held him as if he were a doll." She still feels her emotions "like it was yesterday."

Hospital caregivers made the new family feel secure, but leaving the hospital was frightening. "I was so scared when we brought Jason home. This was both our first child and a child with many health issues."

When Jason came home from the hospital, the demands of the "real world" were stressful for Lee. He had to run his business, help care for Jason, and find a new, accessible home for his family. As life settled down, Lee's experience enabled him to offer installation of accessible bathrooms and ramps through his construction company. People told him, "I'll give you the job because your son has spina bifida and you know something about this."

While the Brandons' extended family was supportive, some of their closest friends backed off or drifted away. Relating to people in the community was also challenging. Priscilla didn't want Jason to feel "different"; she wanted him to go to church, get groceries, and go to the toy store like any other little boy. But occasionally when they went out, small children would point at Jason and a mother would say, "Don't look at him!" Priscilla remembers one such occasion when she longed to tell the mother that her children's curiosity was normal and to tell the children that her son's legs just didn't work the way theirs did. But the mother rushed on.

Afterward, Priscilla sat in the mall, crying. How could she explain her feelings to the mothers she encountered? They didn't know what she was going through. They didn't understand that she also found the blessings in mothering Jason. They didn't know that her son had to try on a dozen shoes to find ones that fit his braces. And they didn't understand that sometimes no shoes would fit and she would sit down and cry. But then Jason would do something wonderful and the scale would balance itself. Positive, fearful, thankful, angry, set apart—all those words described how Priscilla came to feel about the world.

Four years after Jason's birth, Jean was born: a bright, alert little girl who adored her older brother from the start. The siblings had a nurturing, bickering, love/hate relationship with a bit of jealousy on each side, a normal brother-sister relationship. Jean was included in Jason's medical care early on. She was too young to stay home alone, and since her grandparents also went to Jason's appointments, she couldn't stay with them. Jean remembers the whole family piling into the car for clinic visits. Although it was hard for everyone when Jason was in the hospital, Jean never felt left out. "He is not a complainer, and he makes me forget he has spina bifida. He makes me feel proud."

Hospitalizations and surgeries, fourteen in all, were part of their family life. Lee says that having his son hospitalized "is the only thing I've ever cried about. It's harder having your kid in the hospital than a spouse." Priscilla agrees: "You prepare yourself and your child, but when they wheel the child away, you cry." Dealing with the physical and emotional impact of surgeries was difficult. Priscilla recalls Jason asking, prior to one surgery, "Am I going to be able to walk?" and not having a clear answer.

Predictions by medical personnel have been both encouraging and discouraging, and not always accurate, beginning with the geneticist who warned of brain damage that did not occur. Later an orthopedist told them Jason could walk—but the braces didn't work, and he continued to need a wheelchair. There were highs and lows. Some doctors focused mostly on the cost of an operation to determine if it was "worth it" for Jason, but this was balanced by others who based their decisions on what was best for Jason's health and well-being.

Priscilla finds that old memories of Jason's medical issues still "sneak up on her." She recently talked with a mother of a baby with SB, who was told at delivery that her child's SB was very severe with a bleak prognosis of two weeks' survival. Priscilla said all she could think was, "I don't want to hear. Don't talk to me." But the other mother continued: "Another doctor sent us to a special hospital for children. My baby is now ten months and kicking." This sparked the memory of taking Jason to an SB clinic when he was about to enter kindergarten. After the examination, Priscilla overheard the doctor tell the nurse, "I think this kid is slow." When Jason got all sorts of awards at his high school graduation, she wanted to find that doctor and show him how wrong he was.

When Jason was in the eighth grade, he saw a movie in health class about SB. He came home that day and was very quiet. Priscilla could sense his concern and asked him about his day. "We saw a movie," he said and started to cry. "You never told me SB was a birth defect." She explained that when he was conceived her body had no folic acid, adding, "I don't see it as a 'defect.' You were blessed with life."

True to the family's interest in sports, Jason wanted to play baseball. Priscilla and Lee debated whether they should fight to get him on a community team. They tried to avoid the issue, but Jason pushed to apply for a team slot. He was not accepted, but at his request they got him a bat and ball. Priscilla told him, "Just remember that I wanted to be a ballerina but I didn't have the physique or the discipline. I can still have the love and enjoyment of ballet, but it's not for me to do. If you don't make a team, you can still love the sport and play it on your own."

Family activities and vacations are planned so that everyone can participate. Each year the Brandons go to an accessible sports camp located on a beach, where they all experience the thrill of speed and adventure, through active sports like jet skiing and kayaking. In the winter, Lee and Jason are on an adaptive skiing team.

Jason and Jean help out with dinner, fill and empty the dishwasher, and clean their rooms—and Jean washes the dogs and feeds the two pigs, four dogs, and one rabbit of the family menagerie. But Priscilla says schoolwork comes first. Both children set their own goals and make plans to reach them. Priscilla likes it when the kids take on their own projects. Home chores have not been stressed, and Lee thinks that the kids have "skated" on responsibilities.

Jean thinks she and Jason have been protected by their parents in some ways, but that they have also been given enriching life experiences. For instance, she went away to camp by herself, and she learned to surf. She frequently performs, both acting and singing, and writes her own blog. Her parents have supported her in taking these social risks.

Priscilla and Lee have set guidelines for their family, including respect, nonviolence, cleanliness, sharing family meals, church attendance, and going to college. Priscilla says that these are rooted in her experience growing up in a family that was structured and strict with clear expectations.

Religion is a focal point in the Brandons' life. Grandfather Frank set the bar; religion has been his guide for living and raising his children. "You hold religion high, and the kids follow." He is Catholic and attends Mass daily, but he accepts that Priscilla and Lee have joined a Protestant church. "As long as they believe in God, they are okay; they will be good to people and treat them right." Frank believes that God played a role in Jason coming into his family. He once told Priscilla, "God was looking for parents for this child."

For Priscilla, religion helps her stay centered and positive. Her faith is a source of explanation and support to her when she contemplates her son's disability. Although Lee finds it hard to get up early for church, he feels connected to his religious community and beliefs and enjoys being an elder and committee chair.

Priscilla says, "Going to college was a huge accomplishment for Jason. It's normalcy, what every kid wants. He is able to do it." In preparation for taking Jason to college, the Brandons arranged through their state department of rehabilitation for personal care attendants to assist Jason on campus. But when they arrived at his school, there was no attendant for Jason. They learned that the rehabilitation systems of their home state and the one in which the university was located had not coordinated their efforts. Priscilla and Lee worked frantically to resolve the issue but didn't have sufficient time before they had to return to work. Frank, who had accompanied them, stayed on to care for Jason until the two states resolved their differences and attendants were assigned. Lee says it was hard to watch Jason go off to college, but it's another event that makes him think of Jason as a normal kid. "I forget the wheelchair. He still has mental capacities."

Grandfather Frank worries about the future. Although Jason has started college, Frank is concerned about whether he will have full access to educational opportunities at his college and beyond. "We've had to fight even for curb cuts for each school he has attended." And "kids," he believes, "don't earn—they deserve."

# 5

# Grandparents

## Seeing through a New Lens

---

"I look at her waking up of a morning. I sit right outside her bedroom door so she'll see me there and feel safe knowing her granddad is there. We'll build tents and take our flashlight inside. It's given me an appreciation for what we have each day."

—NED, A GRANDFATHER

Grandparents can be parents' ace in the hole, ready to stand in or soothe frayed nerves as necessary. Just as you and your children are expanding your views of what is "normal," grandparents will be rethinking and refocusing their lens to frame a different view of both their able-bodied grandchildren and those who have disabilities. Grandparents usually follow the parent's lead in focusing on each child's abilities without losing sight of the fact that disability can add its challenges. And sometimes grandparents are a step ahead, helping you see your family in a new light.

Even though you are an independent adult, you are still your parents' child, and they want to be in on the highs and lows of your life. Grandparents can help in numerous ways: for example, by being a sounding board for decision making without demeaning you or your parental authority. Their sensitivity—knowing when to offer help and when to stand back—is a key to having a healthy relationship with you and the grandchildren.

Many grandparents have natural radar screens that allow them to assess what their children and grandchildren need from them at the moment. Is this a grandparent's "waiting-in-the-wings" role or a "you're-needed-now!" role? If grandparents miss their cue, you can direct them, letting them know when you need their help and when you don't. Flexibility and communication are critical to managing parent/grandparent roles. This is a learning process for parents and grandparents; you will both get better at communicating your needs and defining your roles over time.

## Grandparents Near or Far

Grandparents may live in the same house as their grandchildren, in the same neighborhood, in the next county, or a continent away. Each distance creates different hurdles for grandparents in remaining a part of their grandchildren's lives. But with a little effort and good communication, emotional closeness between grandparents and grandchildren is possible regardless of geographic distance.

### "In the Vicinity" Grandparents

When grandparents live near you, but not in the same household, they can see you on a regular basis, play with your children, and help out—but still have some distance from the private life of your nuclear family. They can be "on call" for both the up times of your children's lives—dance recitals, holiday concerts, sports events—and down times such as operations and illnesses.

Although you may want your parents to be an active part of your family, you probably don't want to include them *all* the time. But some grandparents who live nearby have trouble respecting the boundaries of their adult children's nuclear family. They drop by without calling ahead, or plan events and dinners without consulting the parents about the fam-

> Grandparents can establish a running thread through interactions with each grandchild. For example, one child loved jokes, so his grandmother bought a book of jokes and had a new one to share during each phone call. A grandfather and his granddaughter loved to talk about the kinds of birds they saw; at holiday time he sent a bird identification book for his granddaughter to keep a record of her bird sightings. Grandparents whose grandchildren love to read can read the same books and talk about them.

> **T** Grandparents may remember when they taught their child to ride a
> bike, running alongside him at first, gradually falling back, and finally
> allowing him to take over. And he did! It is now time for grandparents
> to fade into the background, believing that their child has the ability to
> handle new challenges.

ily's schedule. If this happens, you may feel that you are being treated like a child, as if your parents don't consider you adult enough to make decisions for your own family. You will have to remind them that you are in charge of your own home life and children.

If they feel rejected when you claim your position as head of your own family, it may help to remind your parents that this was the goal of their years of parenting: to see you become an independent person, capable of leading your own life and raising your own children. Grandparents will find that when they recognize your right to make decisions and set limits on their level of involvement, you will actually be more willing to welcome them into your life.

Like Frank Brandon, some grandparents have a larger role in their grandchildren's life, by mutual agreement with their adult children. Ned's granddaughter has spina bifida. He drives her to school and picks her up each afternoon, and he cares for her twenty hours a week while her mother and father are at work.

## "In-House" Grandparents

When grandparents live with their children and grandchildren, the experience can be fulfilling and helpful to all—*if* relationships and roles are clearly defined. "In-house" grandparents regularly witness the workings of their child's nuclear family and, in some ways, become part of the

> **T** When thinking of the way to treat a grown child, grandparents need to
> ask themselves, "How would I treat a friend?" Adult children have the
> same rights to respect, autonomy, and privacy.

☞ If parents are abusive to their children, unable to provide a safe environment for them, or incapable of meeting their basic needs, then grandparents need to step in to protect their grandchildren. Grandparents can report their concerns about parental abuse or neglect to the Child Protection Services Agency in their state. If parents are deemed unfit by the state or voluntarily put their children in grandparents' care, then grandparents who want to do the job may be awarded temporary or permanent custody of the grandchildren.

family system. Yet grandparents are not the parents, and they need to support the parents' rules and roles. Any disagreements with the way parents are dealing with a situation should be discussed adult to adult—and not in front of the grandchildren.

While their adult child may consider grandparents' opinions and advice on parenting, ultimately grandparents must defer to the rules and structure for parenting that their adult child sets for his family.

Finances play a role in the everyday life of every family. Clarifying how household bills and rent or mortgage payments are to be shared by grandparents and adult children is fundamental to the success of multi-generational living. Doing chores or providing services (such as child care) that the family would otherwise need to pay for may be counted as an economic contribution.

Some grandparents may have to live with their children for economic reasons and rely on them for financial assistance; in turn, these grandparents may assume certain responsibilities within the home, such as making dinner or being there for the children after school while parents work. In other families, adult children and their kids get financial help from the grandparents, or live in the grandparents' home in order to make ends

T A live-in grandparent is not the decision maker for the grandchildren unless she has been assigned that responsibility. Her mantra should be, "Better ask my son or daughter if it's alright for me to do that with my grandchild."

meet. Often, adult children (and grandchildren) will repay the grandparents by helping with household chores, driving, yard work, or other things they need. Any of these arrangements can work to mutual advantage—as long as roles and expectations are clear and each generation feels they are gaining something through multigenerational living.

### Faraway Grandparents

For many grandparents who live far away from their grandchildren, keeping in touch is a challenge. Travel is not always possible, but grandparents can connect through telephone calls, e-mail, and Skype, an Internet video chat service. Tech-savvy grandparents may join the world of cell phone texting—increasingly the communication medium of choice for children. Vern enjoys regular "visits" with his son and his family by Skype. Vern lives abroad and can only travel to see his grandchildren every two years, yet he feels very connected to them. He recently heard and saw his grandson's live performance of "Go Tell Aunt Rhodie" on his new trumpet and watched his granddaughter tell him about her first day of ballet school. He likes the spontaneous exchange and a sense of really "being there" in the children's life.

Genevieve, a Canadian, sees her American family a few times each year and talks with them by phone weekly. In this way she keeps up with the latest interests and developments in their lives. Genevieve makes her-

When a grandchild is going through surgery or a lengthy medical procedure, faraway grandparents can stay in touch by texting, e-mailing, or having "face-to-face" talks via Skype. They can send pictures, videos, or links to websites that their grandchildren will enjoy. These interactions divert the grandchild from what he is going through and give the grandparents an opportunity to entertain him, even if not physically present. Ask your parents to create a direct connection with all the siblings so that each feels involved and cared about. When one of your children requires medical attention because of her disability, your focus is on her, and your able-bodied children may feel left out—that's when they can benefit from extra attention from their grandparents.

One grandmother who sees her grandchildren only once a year picks up little gifts she thinks the children might like, wraps them, and puts them in a bag until she has the number of gifts corresponding to the number of days she will visit. Every day each child can choose one of the gifts to open. She does this for her "faraway" grandchildren because she does little things regularly for the grandchildren who live nearer to her. If grandparents don't want to buy gifts, they can find things in nature to share, like a stone from the woods, a beautiful bird feather, some seeds from their sunflowers, or some leftover ribbon or lace from a sewing or craft project.

self more of a presence in her grandchildren's lives by sharing jokes and stories about her pets and her local grandchildren—their cousins. She is also a resource for her daughter and a comfort when needed.

Of course, *actually* being with their grandkids is the ultimate goal for most grandparents. But when families live far apart, visits are so special that sometimes they don't seem quite real. There is so much to pack into a concentrated amount of time that visits can become too intense and exhausting. Scheduling in some rest breaks or time alone will give everyone a chance to relax between family activities. If grandparents can also spend some time individually with each grandchild—to talk, take a walk, or go out for a meal—they will strengthen the bonds they have with each child. Grandchildren will value and remember this special time when they are the focus of their grandparents' attention.

## Grandparents' Supporting Roles
### Support for Adult Children

The American Association of Retired Persons announced in August of 2011 that an increasing number, about 70 percent, of grandparents are stepping in to help with their grandchildren. Grandparents are clearly an important source of support to their children. Their support can be emotional, physical, or financial. Any help from grandparents—when it is wanted by their children—will reduce stress on the family and protect the parents' mental and physical health. Helping also gives grandparents a chance to form closer and more meaningful relationships with their grandchildren.

### Emotional Support to Parents

When a group of grandparents get together, the talk is usually about their grandkids. It's easy to get caught up in the exciting world of grandchildren's lives. Meanwhile, the "sandwich" generation—parents of the aforementioned grandchildren—sometimes feel left out. As one son said to his mother, "What am I, chopped liver?" It's OK for adult children to ask their parents to listen or give them advice. Sometimes you just need your parents to "be there" for you when you are either overjoyed by your child's accomplishments or stressed out by life events.

While grandparents' presence at your child's special events will be welcomed by your children, it's also a way for your parents to show solidarity and support for you. Helen finds that even when her grandkids are disinterested, her children "don't want me to miss any of their kids' activities."

Grandparents can also help by giving positive feedback to their adult children. Receiving appreciation from your own parents or in-laws for ways you treat your spouse, care for your children, or care for yourself boosts your morale and self-esteem. Helen's daughter-in-law, Pili, appreciates it when Helen tells her that her child who has spina bifida "picked the right parents." Pili says, "I owe a lot to my supportive in-laws." When adult children know that their own parents trust them to make wise decisions and to do what needs to be done for their families, they are encouraged to assume their responsibilities with added vigor.

Genevieve trusted her daughter's family to use their personal resources to help her granddaughter meet the challenges of living with OI. She believed they could do whatever was necessary. "Everyone in the extended family had great sympathy for the family and, after the initial shock and disbelief, faced it as a fact of life. Our granddaughter is loved and treated the same as all of our other granddaughters, with no special allowances made other than for her safety." Genevieve's belief in her children's abilities made them feel they had been given "the grandparents' seal of good parenting."

"My Mom knows I can handle this crisis; that gives me the confidence to deal with parenting decisions I make every day."
—Debbie

### Physical Support to Parents

When grandparents are able to give it, physical support (housework, babysitting, chores, and so forth) is invaluable to parents. Earlier, you read about Susie, the mother of four sons, including twins who have physical disabilities. When the twins were 4 years old, Susie had a herniated disc from carrying them up and down stairs in her three-story home. Two years later, the disc ruptured while she was bathing. Her parents, who lived several states away, took the children for six weeks while Susie recovered her strength. Their generous help allowed Susie to rest and recuperate with peace of mind, knowing that her children were in good hands. For the grandparents, this visit was an opportunity to spend "real" 24–7 time with their grandchildren, getting to know each one. This was also a special time for the boys to get closer with their grandparents. Ned also gifts his children with his time when he cares for his granddaughter—and he finds this role a fulfilling part of his life. "She and I are very close."

Grandparents can also help out by structuring playdates or excursions, taking dinner to their grandchild's family, or inviting the children to spend some time at their house while the parents get a rest.

Having a night out is restorative and gives parents a chance to reignite the intimacy necessary to keep their relationship alive. Helen often babysits overnight so her son and his wife can have a complete break from family responsibility. She feels that it's essential for the parents to get a break once in a while, so they can keep their family running smoothly. "The family structure has to work. I don't know what they would have done without us grandparents," says Helen.

Grandparents handy with hammers and nails can help put in ramps or lower light switches to make their child's home more accessible for their grandchild who has a physical disability. A grandchild might ask a grandparent clever with his hands to build a "desk" that fits across his wheelchair for doing work at home or school, or to create custom built-ins in her room, so she can reach her toys and books. Grandparents are prized for the skill they bring to these projects.

### Financial Support to Parents

A family's financial resources are a deciding factor in what they can do for or with their children. If a family has a child who has a physical disability, there is usually more financial stress due to the unanticipated and often rising costs of medications, hospitalizations, doctor's fees, equipment, or home modifications. Some families may have times when it's difficult to meet all their needs.

Grandparents can sometimes help in these situations. Though most grandparents cannot afford to make much of a dent in the mountain of medical costs, they may be able to supplement the family's needs in small but significant ways. Elsie, for example, buys clothing for her grandchildren, which eases the stress on the family budget. "My children are grateful if I buy clothes for the grandchildren. They have never told me to back off—but I tell them to set limits on me if I buy too much." While Elsie's help is valued by her family, she's also aware that her children might feel humiliated or obligated if she gives too much. Her sensitivity and keen ear for their priorities are keys to the close relationship she has with her children.

Grandparents might be able to help with the cost of special equipment (such as a ramped van if the kids use wheelchairs or scooters, or balancing balls for physical exercise) or finance the building of accessible accommodations (like a stair climber up to the second level). This type of help is doubly beneficial as it gives their grandchild more freedom and alleviates muscle strain and fatigue for parents.

Paying for tutoring or activities like music lessons, gymnastics, or art classes is a boon to parents who want to give their children these advantages but can't afford them. Elyse, living far from her family, but understanding their constant struggle to make ends meet, sends them a check before each Christmas to cover the cost of gifts they would otherwise be unable to give their children.

### Support for Grandchildren

Most grandparents want to meet as many of their grandchildren's needs as possible, and they often stretch themselves, giving more than they thought they could. Helen, with grandchildren both able-bodied and who have disabilities, says, "It's a lot of work, but you do what you have to do." She says that meeting the needs of *all* their grandchildren is important. "We don't limit what we do because of my grandson's disability." The family creates ways to incorporate him into the activities they plan for all their grandchildren.

Most grandparents agree that a cardinal rule is to treat all the grandchildren equally. Ned found this important in his own personal development. "I had a hard time being normal in high school when my brother (who had muscular dystrophy) couldn't be. But my parents treated us the same and that always meant so much to me." Ned carries that into his relationship with granddaughter Leeann; he treats her just as he would an able-bodied grandchild.

### Providing Physical Care to a Grandchild Who Has a Physical Disability

Of course, when a grandchild has a physical disability, there are add-on needs—those related strictly to the disability. As a grandparent, it can be challenging—or exhilarating—to learn the new skills involved in caring for that grandchild. "Overnights" with grandparents, special for any grandchild, take on an added dimension when grandparents are learning how to provide hands-on physical assistance and medical care.

Elsie, for example, had to master a few rehab techniques before she could babysit for her grandson Landon. "I took him for ten days so his parents could go on a trip. In preparation I learned how to catheterize and brace him, and get him into his walker. I needed to learn his new enema program, as well as his physical therapy program. I want to be there, to be a good grandma." Elsie enjoys caring for Landon and having some one-on-one time with him, without his parents around. "I like to be fun but also to give him a good example. I find as a grandmother I have time to enjoy him more and I let him try things. He does more than we think he can. He stands on a stool to brush his teeth. I don't stop him from trying."

"My grandfather gave me five cents every time I could walk around the dining room table." —Sam

Elsie and Landon's relationship exemplifies the closeness that can develop when there is the opportunity to care for a grandchild. She has overcome her reservations about meeting his physical needs and feels so comfortable that she can allow him to try things that he has never done before. In the process she has also earned the trust of her children: they know that their son will be well loved and cared for when he is with his grandmother.

### Becoming a Stand-in Parent

When grandparents rearrange their lives to care for their grandchildren, it is usually their choice. For some, like Ned and Frank, helping their grandchildren has become an avocation, which they find personally fulfilling. But some grandparents become sole guardians and stand-in parents for their grandchildren out of necessity. Naomi, for instance, raises her daughter's two boys, one of whom has cerebral palsy, while their mother is in prison. In addition to acting as a parent to her grandsons, Naomi has a job outside the home. She is sustained physically and emotionally by the strong support of her congregation and friends.

Clara is another grandmother who became "mother" to her two granddaughters after her daughter and son-in-law were killed in a car crash that left one of the girls paralyzed. Elina, the girls' aunt, moved in with Clara to share the load of raising them. When the roles of grandparent and parent are fused, relationships with grandchildren can become somewhat murky and complicated. Grandparents in these families become directors, disciplinarians, and schedulers for the children, where before they had primarily been givers of unconditional love and emotional support. Grandparents will often need time to sort out their feelings about these role changes and redefine their relationships with their dependent grandchildren.

When the focus is entirely on the child's needs, grandparents can lose sight of *their* needs. But taking care of self is vital to maintaining the energy and perspective needed to raise children. Support for grandparents can be found through religious congregations, extended family, friends, and sometimes coworkers. An in-depth discussion of custodial grandparents' needs is beyond the scope of this book, but there are other books that can help. In some communities, social service agencies have special services for families headed by grandparents (see the Resources section of this book for other information). Grandparents who find it difficult to maintain their equilibrium with the children or are depressed or overwhelmed might benefit from additional help from a mental health professional.

### Planning for Changes in Grandparents' Ability to Help

Although many grandparents are healthy and active, some will have physical limitations and continue to age as your children grow up. Their ability to help out or to stay emotionally engaged with your children might lessen over time. It's helpful for you and your children's grandparents to anticipate these changes and how they will affect your family, as well as make plans to lessen the impact on everyone.

Helen, for instance, worries about how her son, his family, and she and her husband will all get adequate health care. She says, "The medical costs for a child who has spina bifida can run to half a million dollars! What if my son loses his job? Who will be there to care for *them*? Who will care for *us* when we can't walk? I don't want our children to have to do that." A family meeting with parents and grandparents can help identify specific concerns—such as running out of money in retirement, inadequate health insurance, and finding someone who can help care for your children if grandparents become unable. Then you can begin to make appropriate plans for the future.

## Expanding Grandchildren's Lives

Grandparenting opens up a world of opportunities to do things for and with grandchildren—not just helping, but also adding a layer of experiences to their lives. Parents have an obligation to provide, care for, nurture, love, and educate their children, but "grands" can choose to expand their grandchildren's activities in many directions while building a mutually rewarding relationship with them. Grandparents can add these extra dimensions by enriching their grandchildren's experiences and being present for special moments in their lives.

### Enriching Their Lives

*Being a Companion, Guide, or Explorer*

Ned says, "Being a musician, I appreciate that Leeann can carry a tune." They sing and make up songs, and he works with her hand development, creating gestures to go with the songs. He plays in a band. Leeann loves to listen, sitting in front of her granddad as he plays. Other kids dance with her in her wheelchair; afterward she spends the night with her grandparents. Recently Leeann asked her grandfather, "Why are you wearing white *tennis* shoes?" He replied, "I only wear white cowboy boots when I'm playing in the band." She called out, "Yee haw!" Ned's experience with Leeann combines fun, exposure to music and dance, and inclusion in a community of musicians that enriches both their lives.

Grandparents have unique opportunities to enrich their grandchildren's lives by exposing them to enjoyable and interesting life activities.

Whether letting their grandchildren "teach" them a math lesson or being an enthusiastic fan of their trumpet practice, the older generation can enhance your children's sense of self with their support and praise. Involvement with each grandchild can be "customized" to his interests and abilities; for example, while Hayley loves movies and film stars, her brother Brendan is into geodes. Grandparents can broaden their own horizons by teaming with each grandchild to explore individual interests, which can be enjoyable for all involved.

Esther and her granddaughter Siobhan have become closer through their shared interest in current world events and their "passion about books." Esther says she's followed Siobhan's lead, and they've teamed up "to solve these mysteries together." Siobhan is very curious and often asks probing questions when she's heard an intriguing news story. Esther's assignment is to do the research, tracking down information and answers for Siobhan. Esther relishes this relationship. "It is hard to hug Siobhan because of her spasticity, so we have an intellectual closeness."

Every grandparent has a different twist on favorite activities with his grandkids, reflecting both the grandparent's and grandchild's interests and abilities. Whereas Esther's relationship with Siobhan grows through intellectual activities, Helen likes to explore the outdoors and ride horses with her grandsons. They go to the zoo, fish, and watch wildlife at the pond. Elsie and her grandson like to hike and explore the woods near her home, go boating, bake cookies, and paint pumpkins.

### Handing Down the Story of the Family

Because parents are so busy raising their families, some grandparents take on the task of keeping the family history up-to-date, or delving deep into the past to find ancestral links, providing a foundation of "who we are as a family." This heritage helps children feel more rooted in their family's culture, history, and values—to know that they came from a distinct group of people. Helen passes down the family's lore and cultural heritage by keeping the family photo books and writing Christmas letters telling the story of the family from year to year. She hopes that her grandchildren, though they may not understand the purpose of this now, will be grateful for this history when they get older and learn to appreciate the profound value of family.

### Traveling

If grandparents are financially able—and parents approve—they can take grandchildren on trips by land, sea, or air. This requires lots of advance planning in regard to accessibility and meeting physical needs, but there is information available to make this possible (see Resources section of this book for travel agencies that specialize in trips for people who have physical disabilities). There is nothing like an adventure to bind the generations together. Traveling is a mind-expanding opportunity for children of all ages, and the memories last forever.

### Being Present

"Gram, are you coming to the holiday concert at school?" What your grandchild is really saying is, "Gram, I really want you there to watch me. And I know that you care enough to come." Grandmother's attendance gives the child a sense of belonging to a wider family than just her parents and siblings; it is a lesson in the ways family members support one another. Indeed, a grandparent's presence at the holiday concert is as significant as her presence at the child's bedside when he is in the hospital.

## Grandparenting a Child Who Has a Physical Disability

Just as parents experience "extras" in having a child who has a physical disability, so do grandparents. Challenges and rewards, supporting and being supported, keep grandparents focused on helping their families prepare for the future. Faith, a sense of purpose, and flexibility help grandparents in this family mission.

### Community Support

Helen's way of grandparenting is an extension of how she's always lived and what she's believed. In her childhood community, people expected life to bring ups and downs, and they were prepared. "If someone caught a big fish, we shared it with everyone; our community shared the good and the bad." When an unanticipated event happened, like the birth of a baby who had a physical disability, the community acknowledged it, consoled the family, and supported the family in coping. Sharing whatever came along, positive or not, was a buffer for the family; what happened to one happened to all, and the community was supportive in fair weather and foul. Because Helen was prepared for life by this balanced, down-to-earth worldview, the impact of her grandson's disability was lessened.

### Faith

Elsie's faith is unbroken by the experience of having a grandchild who has a disability. "There is no answer why this happened. There is a reason for everything. Faith has gotten me through so much. If you don't have faith I don't know what you do. This has made us closer. Even if my grandson has a disability, he has a loving family he is part of. No one promised us life would be perfect." Ned's faith is paramount, too. "You have to believe," he says.

While religious faith is central for some grandparents, others put their faith not in a higher being but in their own ability to face life's slings and arrows and in their children's resilience. Marshall believes that events happen randomly, and he can't imagine that there could be a god who would make a child suffer; nevertheless, he has faith that his son and daughter-in-law will raise their children with and without physical disabilities to their full potential.

### A Sense of Purpose

Ned and his wife are more aware of other people who happen to have disabilities since their granddaughter's birth. He struggled when Leeann was born as her disability brought up old feelings of loss for his brother who had muscular dystrophy. "I fought it when Leeann was born. Why? I was handed a little girl. I was bitter over a recent lay-off. I was upset at first but then realized there are many worse off. Now I know it had a purpose—so that I could babysit Leann. When I first started I had to learn how to catheterize and give medicine. When you're the only one there, you do it. I'm loving it." Ned realized that a bad event turned into a meaningful relationship, where he both gives *and* receives love, and in which he is growing in his ability to care.

## Grandparents Adapt and Grow, Too

Grandparenting presents a unique opportunity to reach one's potential as a human being and to develop personal qualities that may have been lacking earlier in one's life—like patience, giving or receiving, being optimistic and hopeful, or being thankful for the "small things." Having a grandchild who has a physical disability among one's other grandchildren provides a whole new perspective on the possibilities in life.

### Generativity

By the time they become grandparents, most people have reached the stepping-stone that Erik Erikson, a developmental theorist, calls the *generative* stage of life. This stage, normally occurring in middle age, is a time when adults continue to develop by being creative and productive in their own lives and by helping the younger generation—in their own family and outside it. Ann expresses this impulse to give and create through her widely known fund-raising efforts for OI, especially "in-door picnics," her signature activity. "I'm making ham, potato salad, everything. It keeps me busy." She has made over seventy baskets of donated goods thus far. "People have been donating to OI through me since Dan was born. As a giver I've had to learn to be aware of other people who give. I have to be thankful to them." But she knows that, even if her grandson had not had OI, she would still be involved. "I like helping people."

### Patience

Grandparents who are type A personalities—hard driving, using every minute to its fullest—may feel stressed when they are out of sync with their children's and grandchildren's slower pace. Grandparents may need to slow down a bit to fit in with the rhythm of life for their grandchildren, especially those who have physical disabilities. Children have their own internal clocks (usually moving at a different rate than adults') and their own agendas and priorities. And grandchildren who have disabilities have internal clocks and agendas *plus* the external schedules of medical or rehabilitation care; they learn to slow down, developing the ability to wait, endure, and be steady. Grandparents need to develop patience, so they can enjoy being in the moment with their grandchildren.

"Having a grandchild who has a physical disability made a huge difference. It made us more patient and understanding. Now we understand the struggles parents with kids who have disabilities go through," says Elsie, whose experience with disability has led to greater patience and tolerance for human differences.

### Giving and Receiving

Some of us are great givers but feel uncomfortable with receiving, perhaps because we feel unworthy or beholden or have little practice. Others are great receivers but do not know when or how to give, or are uncomfortable deciding what another person would like or needs. Grandparents must train themselves to do both well, since grandchildren love to receive gifts—everything from an autumn leaf to a DVD—as well as to give them. Grandparents' reactions to a scribbled "map of your house," a papier-mâché "ball," or a teen's gift of a psychedelic print scarf will be scrutinized for authenticity; grandchildren will be gratified when they determine that grandparents' appreciation is genuine.

For Elsie, in the giving is the receiving. When she knows that her grandson and his parents are coming to visit, she plans the day around their desires, and that brings her happiness. "I enjoy what they give back to me. When the family comes to visit, and I open the door, I hear that little guy squealing from the back seat of the car, 'Nana, get me out of here!' He wants to be with us."

Helen too enjoys the satisfaction of making her family happy. "You have to say, 'I have the time. Let me have the kids.' I want my son and daughter-in-law to have all the time they can find to spend together."

### Optimism and Hope

After resolving some difficult emotional reactions to a grandchild's disability, a grandparent may find that their up-close-and-personal experience of physical disability leads to new levels of optimism and hope—openness to good things, and confidence that one can cope with bad things that come their way. Elsie finds it uplifting that so many people are interested in her life. "People ask about my grandson. People collected money for him. Co-workers bring in things for him. It changed my relationships with others. I am so surprised at how much people care."

## Grandparents Have Their Own Lives, Too

Grandparents today are living different lives than those of preceding generations. Increased life expectancy and advances in technology, as well as their health status, abilities, passions, family needs, and economic conditions, all contribute to the variety of lives they lead. Working life is extended for some, by choice or need, while others opt for early retirement to enjoy travel, recreation, or avocations.

Grandparents have more choices than ever about how to spend their time. While they often choose to play an integral part in their families, their pursuit of individual interests and talents is equally important to fulfillment in the "third act" of life. As their children assume the reins of the family, grandparents are free to let go of being "in charge" and give their attention to other interests.

While raising their own family, they may not have had enough time to follow their own passions. But by the time people become grandparents, they often have more "space" in life to pursue their own passions—career, physical fitness, volunteer work, or hobbies shelved while you, their children, were the main focus. Now, even if grandparents are still fully employed, they can finally say, "It is my time."

In fact, it is vital—for the well-being of grandparents and the entire family—that they remain engaged in the world outside the family. Physical and emotional self-maintenance for grandparents is not selfish; it's wise. When grandparents are taking care of themselves, they will be better prepared to help you and the grandchildren when needed, or just to "be there" for you, in both celebrations and hard times.

The time and effort put into keeping physically and mentally fit are well spent, generating the energy and vitality to tackle what *has* to be done as well as the fun things in life. Building a program of exercise and relaxation and pursuing passions for fulfilling activities or ideas (in addition to being an involved grandparent) are prescriptions for a well-rounded and healthy life.

Elsie and her husband own a small resort on a lake. Begun as a hobby, the resort now has five cottages. They lead a happy, outgoing life, and both place a high value on family. Each also holds down another job, Elsie working at a college. Exercise—walking and running together—is part of their life. Elsie also runs 5Ks, finding them a "stress reliever." Last but not least, they relish being with and helping their four kids and grandchildren. Maintaining a good balance of work, family, couple, and individual activities is their goal.

Inclusive grandparents balance giving with receiving. It takes some time and experience for them to fully develop the ability to respond to their own needs as well as those of their children and their families, especially when one of their grandchildren has a physical disability. It takes a good dose of respect and sensitivity not to intrude on their child's family. But inclusive grandparents are ready, physically and mentally, to step forward when their presence is requested. And for most grandparents, that request for participation is a gift.

# PART III

# Into the Wide World

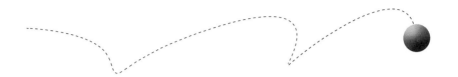

### The Sheridan-Wolfe Family: Two women build their family by adopting children who have complex disabilities and helping them reach their potential

Lynn met her life partner, Jessie, at a wedding, and after some time they began a romantic relationship. Lynn had an adopted daughter, Miranda, who had multiple disabilities, and Jessie had two sons; they knew they were creating a "package deal" when they made their commitment to each other.

Lynn had worked for twenty years as an intensive care nurse and then provided home care when children were discharged from the hospital. In time she became a case manager, assisting children with the transition home and helping families understand their children's needs. Meanwhile Jessie had chosen a career as a counselor, and she discovered a special empathy for children who needed help.

Early on in her work in a large neonatal unit, Lynn observed the number of babies who were not able to leave the hospital because their care was too complex for their families. "I started thinking, 'I love kids. I would want to take these kids home.'" A few years later, Lynn became involved with a family that fell apart. The mother left six children in foster care, went into labor prematurely with the seventh child, and then disappeared after giving birth. "The social worker called me and said, 'Would you take the baby home? You're the only person here who is involved with her.'"

Lynn took baby Miranda home when she was 24 weeks old. Lynn did not feel ready for this, but she felt there was no choice. As they were leaving the hospital, a physician told her, "Don't expect much; she is going to be blind and deaf and she won't walk." Lynn was "floored."

Lynn became a single parent, working full-time. But as soon as she started day care, Miranda began to have medical complications, including recurrent pneumonias. She was suffering from broncho-pulmonary dysplasia (BPD), a respiratory condition that affects some premature babies. Lynn was forced to quit her job because she could not get a home care nurse for Miranda eight hours a day. That was the first time Lynn had to quit work to care for Miranda, but it was not the last.

It was during this time that Lynn and Jessie got together. Jessie became a second mother for Miranda while Lynn became close to Jessie's boys. Erik, the younger of the boys, lived with his father for a year before moving in with his mother and Lynn, going from youngest in the family to the older child role. He didn't fully understand Miranda's disability, but he accepted her. "I just saw her as my new little sister."

At age 3, Miranda was placed in a special school for children who have severe disabilities. In retrospect, Lynn regrets that decision because "kids identify with kids they're around." Miranda seemed more comfortable with other kids who had disabilities because she was in the hospital so much. She was a cute little girl, and Lynn says she learned to play the "poor little thing" role.

At age 7, Miranda transferred to a mainstream elementary school. Her speech was difficult to understand and she used a wheelchair, except in the classroom, where she used her walker. She became a social butterfly, was part of the pack, and was included in all activities with her peers.

Lynn and Jessie were eager for Miranda to have a sister. They were considering a foreign adoption, but then they received a call from a local children's hospital: a family had planned to adopt a baby girl but reneged because of "unknown" medical issues, including some type of brain injury at birth. After meeting baby Siobhan, Jessie and Lynn decided to adopt her. When Lynn's mom, Esther, first heard about Siobhan, she wondered about the wisdom of this adoption; but when Esther met Siobhan, she said, "There is something in there." It took Siobhan some time, but then, Esther says, "she broke out."

Siobhan came home at 2 months of age with a gastrostomy (feeding) tube. Life seemed crazy. When she was 5 months old, the neurosurgeon determined that she had had a stroke while still in utero. Only the part of her brain that controls basic functions such as breathing, swallowing, and motor coordination was damaged by the stroke; early in her childhood, it became clear that her intellect was normal. She had various procedures and ER admissions. Doctors said that Siobhan would need a tracheostomy in the future, but they delayed it until after her second birthday because it would make speaking difficult. Since then, she has had numerous other medical interventions, including the use of a bilevel positive airway pressure ventilator, sleep monitoring devices, and a spinal fusion operation to prevent severe scoliosis.

Erik was exposed to the health care system and his sister's medical needs during those years. He says that Lynn and Jessie "had me help out a little, slowly integrating me into the situation." Erik found that patience was the key to not becoming overwhelmed. "The hospital was not a traumatic event for me." He learned that sometimes his attempts to help could be a hindrance and learned when to back off. "I've never felt my needs diminished by my little sisters' needs. Their needs may be life or death," says Erik.

Erik is grateful to his parents for "showing me how life is, to guide me in the real world." He says that the experiences in his family have been the key to his open-mindedness. "Our norms are different. What is 'normal'? My family is normal. I was young when change came. I expect chaos in life. Whenever everyone is in the box, I've stepped outside and can look back at our world."

During the early years, when the girls lived closer to her, Esther babysat. "I consulted and brainstormed with Lynn because we are both nurses and both like to invent. We think outside the box." She helped to create some of the tools Siobhan uses to control her world. Because Siobhan has spasticity, it is hard to cuddle her, so Esther says they have an intellectual closeness, both being passionate about books and learning. Siobhan has become a very curious teen; she often questions what she hears on newscasts and seeks out further information. Esther is her co-researcher. They like to solve mysteries together. When people refer to Siobhan as a "case" or a "disorder," Esther corrects them: Siobhan is a *person*.

Lynn and Jessie learned that Siobhan's brain was actually "in overdrive"—she was intellectually gifted. At age 3, Siobhan would throw fits if not read to exactly as the words appeared on the page. Later, she used a Gemini voice output system (a communication aid that creates audible speech or readable text for people unable to speak), appropriate for her age. Now, as an adolescent, she uses a computer with PowerPoint and other programs.

Despite her intellectual gifts, Siobhan has not been in a mainstream classroom since second grade. Because of her multiple medical problems, she would need a nurse to assist her in class all day, and the cost was prohibitive. So Siobhan has been homeschooled for many years. Lynn now knows what "learning is" and lets her daughter run with her interests. Recently Siobhan has been studying American history to 1865 and learning about Burke, Locke, and Rousseau; she is itching to learn Mandarin Chinese and Spanish. Her homeschool math and language arts curricula come through a top university program for gifted youth.

Teaching Siobhan has taught Lynn that a parent needs the mind-set of "presuming competence" and looking for ways to help her child accomplish all she is capable of. Lynn's attitude is person-centered: "How do I help Siobhan be Siobhan?" This has required adaptation and creativity. For instance, because of a visual impairment, Siobhan has difficulty seeing black ink on white paper; they have found that orange- or peach-colored plastic overlays cut the glare and make reading easier. When working on an adaptation, Lynn tries to use what is commercially available, but sometimes she has to improvise. When Siobhan needed a way to hold down her paper while writing or painting, Lynn, with Esther's help, improvised a tool combining a cabinet door latch, an old computer mouse, some buckshot, and industrial Velcro!

When Siobhan took a class in conflict resolution at a local university, she needed a way to participate in class and gain the professor's attention. Lynn and Jessie rigged a bicycle light to her wheelchair with a touch switch to turn it on. As Jessie says, "If a tool is not out there, how can you help your child be all she can be? You can't stop at 'No, it doesn't exist.'"

With Erik having graduated from high school and working, Miranda in a vocational life skills program, and Siobhan progressing, Jessie and Lynn have recently taken in another little girl, Annette, just 4 years old. Annette had a significant disability; she had been institutionalized and had never used a bathroom, communicated, or even sat upright. But Lynn saw the "intelligence in her eyes" and knew she would fit into their family.

Annette recently had an allergic reaction that resulted in a hospital stay overlapping with her birthday. Lynn took party horns in for every staff member so they could all help celebrate this big event in her life. "People change their behaviors when a child is seen as competent, having opinions, likes and dislikes. Sometimes parents have to lay out those expectations" and show the way.

Lynn says, "I always wanted children. This is the journey of my life. All the pieces come together. I don't think about the physical dynamics of the needs of the girls and my aging. I wasn't planning on this latest little 4-year-old munchkin. And Siobhan is going to be tall; I'm five feet four. Siobhan needs complete physical support."

Mothering the three girls has helped Jessie learn to show compassion, and she has come to experience more compassion for herself, as well—especially since she was struck by lightning a few years ago and can no longer work. She is "different than before. When working for my BA I didn't open a book and got all As. I was struck by lightning while working on my MA; I couldn't do it. I accept myself for where I am."

Lynn's professional background has helped in her parenting, but if people assume she has a huge knowledge base, they are sorely mistaken. Lynn says the secret is to know how to ask questions. "It has to be in language people understand; you need to gauge that understanding. I am often asked by professionals and other individuals if I can find some resources or documents. I find they are not asking questions in a way that will get the answers they need. This is a good skill I learned in childhood: find another way to ask the question."

Lynn remains sensitive to the issues she recognized in high school, when she first worked with families of children who have disabilities: the lack of communication between families and educational systems, and the need for competent medical care, a family support network, and getting people to listen.

Lynn and Jessie work together to support each other and their children. "We couldn't be without the other person. We are each other's safety sounding board. We are a team, willing to drop everything, to be with the child in the space where they have to be; that comes from having to be there in the ER *now*. We feel compelled to fix, give an answer. We both have the ability to see a puzzle piece, change the interlocking one around, move."

Both find bits of time to replenish themselves, Jessie through Native American spirituality and Lynn through the refreshing practice of Tibetan chanting. "You have to find yourself," even if you can't leave your kids to go on vacation.

Lynn says that for her and Jessie, as it is for other parents of kids who have severe disabilities, it's difficult to imagine what lies ahead. "Families are struggling so hard to just get through the day to day that they can't venture a thought about the future, potential, and possibilities." The future may evoke fear for many families; some are grieving the loss of their child's normal developmental stages and the inability to be parents without providing medical care. Parents need help dealing with grieving and with their feelings about having to cause pain and discomfort in caring for a child's physical needs. Other issues Lynn sees affecting parents are the sense of isolation, advocacy efforts being misunderstood, the psychological impact of "well-intentioned" comments and actions, and the problem of meeting the child's need for touch and physical closeness because of the child's paralysis, spasticity, or rigidity.

What would Lynn and Jessie be doing if they hadn't taken this journey? "Probably working twelve-hour shifts, not having found the everyday human piece of life," says Lynn.

# 6

# Opening Doors to Inclusion

- - - - - - - - - - - - - - - - - - - - - - - - - - - - - - - - - - - - - - - - - - - - - - - - - - - - - - - - - - - - - -

"I worry about what my daughter's life will be like when she grows up."

—MIA, THE MOTHER OF

A DAUGHTER WITH OI

"Most teens 'take' independence; adolescents with disabilities may have to be 'given' independence deliberatively."

—RHODA OLKIN, PhD,

PSYCHOLOGIST

## Preparing to Launch

Parenting takes so much energy, love, time, fortitude, and creativity that while you're doing it, it's hard to imagine a time when your full-time involvement will no longer be necessary. Of course, parenting never really ends, but as your children mature and gain independence, your role can become more supportive and less directive. If you are like most families in our society, your ultimate goal as a parent is to see your children become independent and able to leave the nest. Some young adults who have physical disabilities can live independently without any special assistance, but others need help with household chores, transportation, moving about, or activities of daily living (showering, eating, or dressing). If your child needs regular help with these activities, you may be worried about whether she can make it on her own. This chapter explores how you can prepare your child who has a physical disability to be *socially and psychologically independent* even if he needs some help from others to accomplish physical tasks.

## Laying the Groundwork

Launching your children—whether able-bodied or having disabilities—from the comfort and safety of home will be more successful when everyone in the family has envisioned their "release" into the wide world and prepared for this early on. As we have seen, parents do this by gradually exposing their children to greater levels of responsibility and to experiences that build their character and support their relationships with peers. Parents lay the groundwork for their children's eventual independence by fighting negative stereotypes, communicating their expectations for competence, instilling values, and reinforcing character traits that will help their children cope with the ups and downs of life. Additionally, parents can help their children gain access to educational, social, and recreational activities throughout childhood and tap into resources that will support them once they leave home.

### Combating Stereotypes and Negative Attitudes

"They just don't get it!" As the parent of a child who has a physical disability, you've probably had this thought hundreds of times. You have no doubt met some people who demean your child (or you) with condescending words and attitudes, sometimes unintentionally. They think that your child's disability defines her as a person—and assume you do, too. While you see your child as whole and perfect as she is, others may focus on her orthopedic appliances—and lose sight of the child who's using them.

When Pili encounters these attitudes toward her child, she feels "set apart, fearful, a little angry about the way people look at my son or talk about him. I cry and move on." These are the people who give *sympathy* (they assume that a person who has a disability is inferior, and that *they know* what the person needs) when it would be more helpful to express *empathy* (seeing the person who has a disability as an equal, and trying to understand her inner experience). One mother remembers grocery shopping with her daughter who walked with crutches. An older man approached her, saying, "Bless you!" and handed her a card with a religious text promising miracles. The mother was not interested in this man's sympathy; she handed the card back, saying, "Save this for someone who needs it."

There is a little mental trick to distinguish between empathy and sympathy. We call it "the altitude of attitude" because it has to do with the way the recipient of concern feels afterward. Do you feel that the person is looking up to you as if you are a saint in the sky? Do you feel that you are being looked down upon, like a child getting a pat on the head? Or do you feel like you are on the same level, knowing that the other person would "shoot the breeze" with you or tell you the latest joke? This understanding is one to be tucked into your child's toolbox as well; it can help her recognize and gravitate toward people who "get it," and/or to read people more accurately and choose whether or not to educate them or try to change their attitudes.

Liz believes that parents can model positive attitudes for others. "You need to establish the pattern by treating your child who has a physical disability like all other children. People will take their cue from you." Another mom, Kelsey, says that her daughter's disability "is obvious. I used to care what people think and say, but not anymore. Now I just get my daughter out to do whatever girls her age are doing."

Liz and Kelsey have learned to stop asking whether their children *should* do a particular activity, or even whether they *can* do it. Instead, they seek out a variety of life experiences and activities that can enrich their children's relationships with peers and boost their self-confidence and skills. Then they find out *how to make it possible* for their children to take part. By making sure their kids share experiences with their able-bodied peers, Liz and Kelsey give the message—to their kids and others—that their children are "regular kids," neither on higher nor lower planes than their classmates and friends.

### Communicating Confidence in Your Child

Communicating confidence in your children's ability to cope, to thrive, and to achieve adult goals is essential to encouraging their dreams. You can open doors for your child by giving her the message that she has the potential to achieve her goals.

One young woman, who developed quadriplegia from a spinal cord injury at age 12, recalls that right after her injury, "I wanted no part of the life I was enduring and selfishly tried to drag my family into the misery that was overwhelming me. But they refused to go along, challenging me to reach for more than I was willing to believe was possible."

Sam, on the other hand, wishes his parents had praised him more when he was a young boy living with the effects of polio. Sam, now a grandfather himself, advises parents to "pump up your child's self-esteem. Don't give up on the child; they look to their parents to see if they're valuable."

Donny is 13 and has a disorder affecting muscle and joint growth. When he worries about what he can do when he grows up, his parents remind him that his abilities and skills can change as he grows. They encourage him to think about a wide range of possibilities in life.

Recognizing and reinforcing your children's unique assets—intellectual abilities, character strengths, or special talents—is another way to build their confidence. Focusing on your child's positive attributes and abilities can also help him learn to speak up for himself and guide him toward a career or life plan that puts his best qualities to use.

Lynn and Jessie's daughter has multiple physical disabilities but is intellectually gifted, and they have encouraged her intellectual strivings. "She's an awesome student," says Lynn. From her experience teaching her daughter, Lynn has come to appreciate "what learning really is. . . . I let her go with her interests. She reads philosophy, politics, and history books. She's in a gifted youth program and takes math and language courses taught by an Ivy League college. I've learned not to sell her short!"

Some character traits, while "difficult" in the younger years, may help a child strive for independence and self-determination when she is older. Diane recognizes this in her daughter, Rochelle, who has OI. Always "strong willed and determined" as a toddler, Rochelle needed to be watched carefully to prevent accidental injuries. But now that Rochelle is almost a teenager, Diane can see that these character traits "will serve her well in the long run."

### Balancing Dreams and Limitations

Encouraging your child to find a balance between "thinking big" on the one hand and realistically sizing up his abilities on the other will help him make career plans and choose hobbies in which he can be successful. Pointing out that everyone is limited in some ways and sharing the history of your own life choices and compromises can sometimes be helpful.

Priscilla Brandon says that she always told her son who has spina bifida "to follow his dreams." However, "when he said he wanted to be a baseball player, we said, 'Let's get a bat and a ball—but remember that I wanted to be a ballerina, but I didn't have the physique or the discipline. I can still have the love of ballet and enjoy it, but it's not for me to do. Just remember if you can't be on a baseball team, you can still love the sport and play it on your own.'"

Priscilla's example works for both able-bodied children and those who have disabilities. As Rhoda Olkin points out, most people don't have the height to play professional basketball or the flexibility to be an acrobat, but neither do they "dwell on these 'limitations.' We all get what we get and then cope with what we've got."

Parents may want to err on the side of letting their kids have their dreams, even if they seem unrealistic at first. If you give your children the opportunity to work toward their dreams or goals, they will find their own "ceiling" through trial and error. More than likely, they will get frequent "reality checks" from other people who point out their inability to meet certain goals—and they will have to make adjustments. But when you listen to your child and encourage her to think creatively and fully explore her interests, she may find a way to realize her dream, in some fashion. Children whose interests and talents are valued by their parents (or other adults) may be able to use their intellect or personality traits to pursue careers or hobbies that would otherwise be closed to them because of their physical disabilities. This is one way to reach the middle ground between dreams and limits.

Sam says he "had great teachers" who saw his talents and potential and who helped open doors for him. "I wanted to be a lacrosse player, but I couldn't play sports, so I became the scorer and manager and did the team's laundry." As a young adult, Sam's intellect, good communication, and social skills allowed him to "identify bridges, key into society, establish presence, give value, and find a way to connect with others." He built a successful, multifaceted career, got married, had a family, and contributed to society at large.

Eliza, a young adult who has cerebral palsy (CP), comes from a family that values academic achievement. Although Eliza has mobility limitations,

"Don't treat your child differently just because she has a disability. If she wants to do something, let her try. Give her room, space; let her breathe."
—Felicity, a young woman with paraplegia

she is a good writer and has used her talents as the editor of her campus newspaper. She wants to become a newspaper or book editor after acquiring a graduate degree in English. Eliza sees herself "living a good life on my own, not relying on my parents."

### Providing Positive Role Models

Donny's dad says that, at 13, "he's getting to an age where it would be eye-opening for him to meet some adults who also have a disability. It would help him see what other people are capable of and expand his horizons."

Finding positive adult role models for your children (besides yourself) can expose them to different interests, hobbies, and occupations. For all children, having adult role models from different backgrounds, including both able-bodied adults and those who have disabilities, leads to appreciation of diversity, debunks stereotypes, and increases tolerance. But when a child is the only person in his family who has a physical disability, exposure to adults who have disabilities may be especially helpful for him. Ideally, when introducing your children to an adult who has a disability, you want to choose someone whom you admire and respect as a total person—not only because of his or her success in living with a disability—and who can be a role model for your able-bodied children as well. If you don't have a friend who has a disability, you may need to introduce your child to disability organizations or recreational events where adults who have disabilities are active.

Lance, a high school wheelchair athlete, was unique in his school. His same-age peers were able-bodied teenagers whose opportunities for success in athletics were much more varied than his. When Lance started traveling with a wheelchair cycling team, he met adult athletes who had disabilities, who introduced him to the excitement of competitive cycling and provided role models for success as a differently abled cyclist.

### Giving Your Child Responsibility

Having consistent expectations for responsibility instills confidence and is crucial in preparing your child for independent adult roles—work, parenthood, and managing a home. Along with insisting that their children do for themselves, some parents find it helpful to remind their kids that they won't be around to "be there" for them forever. This can spark a series of discussions about the habits and responsibilities the children must cultivate to be independent and a realistic exploration of the kinds of resources and assistance they will need after leaving home.

Candy, a college sophomore who has CP, says, "I am who I am today mostly because my parents refused to baby me. They didn't spoil me or treat me like I couldn't do anything. They made me do what I could. My dad's motto was, 'Seize the day!' They expected me to try new things and work hard." Candy sometimes got angry when her parents wouldn't help her, but now she thinks she's a stronger person because they made her do everything she could for herself. "My parents made me accountable—just because I'm in a wheelchair didn't mean I could get off easy on responsibilities." Candy's mom also encouraged her to go to social events, telling her, "I won't always be here to hold your hand—you need to make friends your own age."

Like Candy's mom, Liz expected her daughter Janet, who has spina bifida, to have responsibilities as she was growing up—to help care for her younger sib, practice her musical instrument, do some light housekeeping chores, and cook dinner once a week. But Liz says that, even though Janet was "determined to be independent and go to college, she wouldn't always take care of herself." Her mom sent Janet for counseling as a teen, to help her become more responsible for her own physical care.

Sometimes it's hard for parents to keep up consistent expectations for their child who has a physical disability. It's tempting to cave in, when you see your child struggling. Liz notes that it took "patience and stamina" for her to "stick with the program" with Janet, "but the result was worthwhile," as Janet is now an independent, married woman.

Sam's family also assigned chores for him as well as his able-bodied brothers. "I had work to do—a lot was expected of me." These responsibilities contributed to his strong work ethic and self-confidence, which served Sam well as an adult with a challenging career and a family.

Giving your child responsibility in any area of life will help build his belief in himself. Although she may have only a small range of responsibilities at home, your child's definition of herself as a *responsible person* will tend to spread into other areas of her life. As they grow, kids who were given responsibilities at home will be more comfortable accepting the variety of responsibilities they need to take on adult roles in the future.

For example, older siblings who help care for younger ones—babysitting, driving them to school, or helping them with homework—learn important adult skills, such as safety awareness, being on time, and communicating their expertise to others. These can help them succeed in college, on the job, and when they become parents. Summer jobs for teenagers, whether they are paid or volunteer, give them another chance to increase their range of responsible behavior. Although jobs are harder to find for teens who have disabilities, you may be able to help your teen find volunteer or paid work in a friend's business, at a local hospital or non-profit organization, or in his or her high school's office or library. Many parents pay their teens for babysitting younger sibs or doing other chores around the house. This is another way to reinforce their sense of responsibility and prepare them for adulthood.

### Allowing Your Child to Take Risks

Helping your children assess and take some risks and gradually take on responsibility for the consequences of their risk taking is another way to work toward independence. These risks can be social, emotional, or physical. All children benefit from "stretching" themselves by risking rejection in an attempt to make a new friend, ask for a date, apply to a difficult academic program, or participate in a sport where there is a small risk of getting hurt. Parents find it particularly daunting to let their children who have physical disabilities take risks, especially when bodily harm may result. But, like all children, these kids need to explore the limits of their bodies, minds, and emotions—and find their own comfort zone for acceptable risk.

Jon recalls that he never rode a bike as a child, because of the risk of falling and breaking a bone. But he was allowed to make this decision himself. "I was pretty intuitive about what would hurt. I wasn't stopped from doing things by my family." Jon believes that "kids need to do normal things" and that parents shouldn't be so protective that they prevent them from doing any activity that poses a small degree of risk. Jalah, Jon's mom, who also has OI, agrees with him that "you need to let your child set their own limits."

The same applies to social and emotional risks. When your daughter who uses a wheelchair wants to ask a boy she likes to the junior prom, she is risking the pain of rejection, just like her able-bodied sister or friends.

But only by asking does she have any chance of success! You can help boost her confidence and, if she does not succeed at first, encourage her to try again. It's important to remember the old saying "nothing ventured, nothing gained."

### Teaching Your Children to Ask for Help

Teaching your child to ask for help might seem like an exercise in dependence, but knowing when and how to ask for help is actually critical to the psychological and social *in*dependence of all children. Children who are not encouraged to ask for help when they need it—or who are pressured to "be strong"—may reject assistance and suffer needlessly.

Sam had polio as a child but was never told what was wrong with him or what to expect. He learned to "fight" his disability, hoping "others didn't see me limping so they wouldn't pity me. I wouldn't dream of being a burden. I didn't use assistive devices until I was 45 years old."

Had Sam been given a more positive message about the use of assistive devices (such as his crutches) as tools for independence and freedom, he might have walked more efficiently or with less pain.

Knowing when and how to get help in a variety of situations (not just with physical activities) is a basic part of becoming an adult. For example, when your able-bodied son is away at college and starts failing a math class, you won't be there to help him. To solve this problem, he needs to find out where he can get help on campus—perhaps from a tutor, teaching assistant, or a fellow student—and he needs the social skills to explain his need, ask for help, and use it most effectively. When your child has a physical disability, he is likely to need the same types of help as his able-bodied peers. But if he also needs physical assistance on a regular basis, learning how to ask for help will be essential to his ability to function without parents.

As a parent, you can help your growing child develop an awareness of what she can do on her own and what she needs help with and make sure she has an accurate understanding of her physical and medical care needs. You can "reframe" your child's ability to ask for help as a sign of his increasing knowledge, competence, and maturity. You and others who help your child while she's growing up can teach her how to direct her care, so that by the time she is an adolescent, your child will be able to tell another person exactly *what* she needs done and exactly *how* to do it—

for example, the methods used for bladder care or for safe transfers in and out of her wheelchair.

Of course, you also need to teach your child when it is *not* appropriate or necessary to ask for help and encourage him to do as much as he can reasonably do for himself.

### Special Considerations for Launching a Teen Who Has a New Disability

When your child acquires a physical disability in the teen years, you have less time to prepare him for living successfully as an adult and coping with his disability. Although a teenager already has more life experiences and social connections than a child who acquires a disability in elementary school, it may be hard for him to leave the nest so soon after experiencing this life-changing event.

This is partly because, in most families, control gradually shifts from parents to child during the teen years—but this process is delicate and easily disrupted by stressful events. When a physical disability unexpectedly enters the picture, both teens and parents experience feelings of loss and anxiety that can interfere with the progress of this normal transition. Families tend to revert to an earlier mode of interacting—with parents grabbing the opportunity to take back control and teens taking advantage of the chance to be relieved of difficult responsibilities.

Felicity is a young woman who has paraplegia from a spinal cord injury at 19. After her injury, Felicity recalls that she "regressed in my parents' eyes." Her parents started treating her more like a child than a teenager about to leave home, constantly nagging her to "take my medicine, push myself harder, do more exercises!" rather than allowing her to be responsible for herself.

Ashley had a similar experience. She had a car accident at 17 and developed weakness and difficulty walking, ultimately diagnosed as a spinal cord injury. Because her family felt sad about her accident and disability and wanted to protect her, "they treated me like a child."

If you can resist the temptation to treat your injured teen as if he had suddenly become a toddler again, he will be more likely to continue on his course toward psychological and social independence, despite his physical impairments. When you help your teen with her physical care, you may be reminded of how you cared for her in early childhood and the tender, protective emotions you felt back then. But it's important to remember that your child is still the same teenager he was before his injury—intellectually, socially, and emotionally. While you may need to help her or to "cut her some slack" with physical chores or jobs she can't do as efficiently (or at all), you can help your teen to maintain her steps toward social and psychological maturity—and to keep herself moving forward.

## Making a Plan

By the time they are teenagers, each of your children should be putting together a practical plan (with your assistance) for venturing out into the world beyond the family—to college, vocational training, work, or another productive adult role—and becoming independent in managing daily life activities, health needs, and social life. This plan should include vocational goals (such as getting an education, a job, or a volunteer position), social goals (such as dating, living with friends or roommates, traveling, or getting married), and recreational goals (such as involvement in sports, arts, or hobbies), as well as an assessment of the economic, social, and other resources your child needs to achieve those goals.

"Slow down and get to know your children individually. How can you support and help them build their individuality? Strategize, triage, and help them reach what they want." —Mary, a mom

When your child is a teenager, you should answer these questions together: What is my child's plan for the immediate future? Where does she see herself five or ten years from now? What skills and resources does he need to make his goals possible? If one of your children has a physical disability, you may have an additional layer of questions: Will my child need physical assistance from others (such as a PCA or part-time aid) in order to live away from home? Will he need special accommodations or technological aids at college or in the workplace? Does she need disability-specific education on sexuality or birth control? Once you have answered these questions, your child's plans for the future will start to take shape. Then you can set about finding the resources and providing the specific tools she needs to reach her goals.

## Getting Off the Ground

Most teenagers begin to plan for their immediate post–high school future by talking to their parents and scouting the Internet to find the most compatible colleges or job placements. Arthur, a young father who has benign congenital hypotonia, points out the benefits of "seeking the counsel of other people in making choices about education, and what to focus on." Teachers, guidance counselors, peers, clergy, and extended family members can act as "consultants" to help you and your teenager figure out the best educational or vocational path.

Most teenagers have no major health problems, and just making sure they have health insurance through their parents, school, or employer is sufficient to send them on their way. But for a teenager who has a physical disability, relocating for college or work may necessitate finding a new doctor or health care team who has expertise in their particular disability. As importantly, these teenagers, especially if they have acquired a disability recently, need to become familiar with laws that protect their rights to equal education and employment and with the resources (such as offices for students who have disabilities, which exist on most college campuses, and departments of vocational rehabilitation, which exist in every state) that can ensure they get the best education or training.

### Landing Gear: Tools for Independent Living

Getting your child ready for success "on the ground" requires motivation, determination, and *information*! Familiarity with resources is essential to open the doors of opportunity for your child. In the rest of this chapter, we discuss how you can help your child participate in the essential activities of adult life that parents of able-bodied children take for granted—social and recreational pursuits, education, vocational training, dating and intimate relationships—and teach them to manage their own medical and health needs. Along the way, we give some examples of parents using their skills as public advocates to improve access and inclusion for their own kids—helping others in the process.

### Social Life and Recreation

"Lance has had one best friend since fourth grade," says his mom, April. But he has not been included in many social activities with his peers.

"He doesn't get invited to parties; he has never been to a birthday party," says April. Lance and his parents have put more energy into his involvement with athletics as a wheelchair cyclist, but even in this arena, Lance's social connections have been mostly with adults, not other teens.

Kids like Lance, who use wheelchairs or crutches, face architectural barriers to attending birthday parties and other social events, but attitudinal barriers are more likely a factor when a child who has a disability is never even *invited* to a birthday party. How can you help your kids get included in the social life of their peers? Some parents take the lead, by regularly inviting their child's classmates to their home (or another accessible location) for playdates, parties, and sleepovers. Others talk to the parents of their child's classmates or teammates and answer questions about their child's disability, to put them at ease. If your child is invited to a friend's party at a location that is not accessible, you can suggest an alternative venue that is. But when that is not possible, you might be able to "bump" your child up the steps in her wheelchair.

> "The accessibility issue is big. It's like you don't belong and in general things aren't made for you." —Pili, a mom

Teaching and modeling social skills for your child, such as how to start up and how to take turns in a conversation, will make him a more attractive playmate or friend. If you have helped her develop varied interests—so she has something to share with other kids—your child will have an easier time joining in with social groups. Because kids who have disabilities often have extra "appendages," like wheelchairs or crutches that draw negative attention, it's helpful (especially in the teen years) for them to dress according to the latest fashion trends and express themselves through clothing and accessories that they and their friends think are cool.

It's also important to talk to your child about how things are going with his peer group and friends. Bullying has become an unfortunately common problem for school-age kids, and your child who has a physical disability may be picked on or bullied at school and need encouragement to talk about it and to let you help him find solutions. Or he may be trying to connect to other kids through inappropriate means, such as becoming the aggressor in school or on the playground. He might try to get attention by being the class clown but never make friends with an individual classmate. You can work directly with your child's teacher to create a more

"There are no
other kids in
wheelchairs
in my school
besides me. I feel
okay about it;
I have lots of
friends and go
everywhere with
them. —Christy,
age 16

accepting atmosphere in her classroom, to encourage social interaction between your child and her classmates during recess or team projects, and/or to help your child learn better ways to initiate social contacts and make friends.

It may also help to explore places for your child to meet and socialize with peers, outside of school. Taking music, art, or swimming lessons; joining 4-H, the Y, or a scouting troop; and going to summer camp are some examples.

The earlier you begin supporting your child's social relationships with peers, the better. Friendships and recreational activities help kids develop essential social and communication skills. When your child has a variety of social opportunities early in life, he is more likely to develop mature social skills and have more enjoyable relationships as an adult. Encouraging your teenagers—whether able-bodied or who have disabilities—to participate in social activities and develop friendships will help them build the social support they need to make their transition to independence.

Encourage your kids to be a part of whatever their peers are doing—at school, at their community center, or in their neighborhood. Creating a skit for a talent night at school, going to the school dances with a group of kids, or asking a girl for a date may be challenging for your child, but with your help, he can find a way to participate.

When transportation to special events (like a scouting trip) is a problem, your child may be able to find a sponsor to provide an accessible bus or van. If he can travel in a car but cannot drive, he may be able to get a ride with another teen or a parent.

"Where play
dates are
concerned, yes,
it's a challenge as
people tend to
forget that she
has OI because
there are no
visual reminders
of her issues.
Rochelle has
hurt herself just
jumping on
beds." —Diane

Finding recreational activities and sports that work for your child who has a disability can sometimes be challenging. As we have shown throughout this book, many kids who have disabilities participate in swimming, baseball, cycling, horseback riding, skiing, and other sports, either with or without special equipment or accommodations. Many recreational organizations, for example, the Boy Scouts, Girl Scouts, 4-H, and YMCA programs, are open to children who have physical disabilities. These kids deserve equal rights to be part of mainstream groups and teams. Parents sometimes have to step in to advocate for their inclusion. When joining an inte-

### Advocating for Inclusion

When Judy saw the obstacles her son faced after becoming a wheelchair user, she was determined to open up the world to him. After tackling the accessibility problems in her own home to allow him more freedom to get around in the house, Judy began to identify barriers in and out of their neighborhood. Armed with the knowledge of what was needed, she searched funding sources in the county and advocated at public meetings for curb cuts to be placed at various intersections, so that her son could travel from block to block in his wheelchair without assistance. Ultimately, Judy campaigned for a playground in her neighborhood; its universal design allowed both able-bodied kids and those who have physical disabilities to play together. Judy became a powerful role model for her son; as a teenager, he started his own advocacy website for people who have physical disabilities.

### Advocating for Access

Tony's son relied on the para-transit system to get around, since they couldn't afford a wheelchair van. Tony was fed up with frequent bus delays and cancellations that caused his son to arrive late to class parties and Saturday swim sessions at his local pool, which were his main oppor-tunities to socialize with friends and meet girls. Tony joined his county's commission for people who have disabilities and led a campaign to reform transportation services for citizens who have disabilities in his city. With an increase in the number of para-transit buses and more frequent stops, Tony's son and others relying on the system gained better access to their favorite social and recreational activities.

grated ability group is not feasible, your child can gain access to a variety of activities through organizations devoted specifically to adaptive sports, recreation, and camping experiences. (Many of these are listed in the Resource section of this book.) For some kids, this feels like segregation and stigmatizing; but for those who are comfortable joining in, it feels liberating. You should discuss this with your kids and honor their prefer-ences and reasoning. If your child needs such extensive assistance that only a special disability program will enable his participation in sports or recreation, it is probably beneficial for him to give it a try. Being with other kids who have physical disabilities is a supportive experience for some kids and can potentially bolster your child's self-image and give him perspective on his particular disability.

### Education

ACCESSIBILITY Several important federal laws protect the rights of people who have disabilities and ensure access to education and vocational opportunities. The Individuals with Disabilities Education Act of 1990, which was revised in 1997, requires schools to provide a free and appropriate education to all children who have disabilities. School systems must make reasonable accommodations (that is, modifications in the way children are taught, the amount of assistance they are given, the technologies they use to do their work, and so forth). Children who have physical disabilities cannot simply be sent to a "special school," but must be included in mainstream education (regular classrooms and schools) whenever possible. This is consistent with the concept of raising children in the "least restrictive environment" and allows them to share as fully as possible in the same educational opportunities that are available to able-bodied children. Schools must be made physically accessible to children who have disabilities, or if they cannot be fully accessible, then accommodations must be made. For example, if your child who uses a wheelchair goes to a public high school with multiple floors, there must be an elevator, or the school must offer any class your child wants to take on the first floor of the building.

Some parents of children who have physical disabilities choose to do homeschooling, sometimes for the same religious, practical, or philosophical reasons that parents homeschool their able-bodied children. While homeschooling allows parents to individually tailor their child's educational program and avoids certain hassles, like transportation to school, it may make it even harder for your child to form friendships or learn the social skills he will need to live independently as a young adult. (If your child has been attending public school and develops a new disability, he may qualify for home tutoring through the school system during his period of recovery from acute illness or trauma.)

ACCOMMODATIONS Your child's physical disability may not be obvious to the school, especially if she is able to walk without assistance. Perhaps she has weakness in her hands and needs to use a computer for writing or a tape recorder to "take notes" in class. Or perhaps he has difficulty with bladder control and needs permission to use the bathroom on demand. These issues—and any other special needs related to your child's disability—should be brought to the attention of the school, so your child can be evaluated for accommodations. The school is obligated to evaluate your child's abilities, disabilities, and medical needs (sometimes using outside experts, such as your child's doctor or physical therapist). Within thirty days of the school's deciding that your child is eligible for services, they will prepare an Individualized Educational Plan (IEP). This written document describes your child's needs, based on professional evaluations and your input as a parent, and details the school services or accommodations that will be provided to meet them. Parents are included in the initial and subsequent IEP meetings; discussion of the plan and your agreement with the recommendations are necessary for implementation. If you and the school cannot come to an agreement about what your child needs, you may seek independent medical evaluations, use mediation services, or ask for a hearing. The IEP is reviewed periodically and can change over time as your child's needs change; keeping the school informed about changes you believe are necessary is vital to the process.

HELPERS, ATTENDANTS, AND AIDES Kids who have physical disabilities and need physical assistance or accommodations at college can usually find resources on campus. Almost all colleges in the United States now have an office on disability to serve students who have special needs. While there is no obligation to report a physical disability during the application process, students who are admitted to a college should contact the disability office as soon as they enroll—especially if they will need regular assistance (such as a personal care assistant, a reader, a person to help transport them on campus, special access to elevators). Early planning will help avoid situations where your child is stuck in his dorm room without an aide to get him ready for class, or has to spend the first two weeks of the semester "bumming" rides from classmates who can push his wheelchair to classes across campus. As Arthur points out, it's important to "accommodate the disability without making it a distraction."

In some cases, your state's department of vocational rehabilitation (see the next section) will work with your child's college to arrange for a personal care attendant (PCA), ensure that your child has access to dormitories and classes, or provide other types of special assistance. For teens like Jason, who has spina bifida, a PCA is a necessity at college—or anywhere he goes without parents around to provide his care.

Kevin, who has quadriplegia from a car accident, emphasizes the importance of hiring one's own attendant, rather than relying on a family member to provide personal care. If your child needs a PCA, learning how to negotiate his relationship with the attendant and to hire, fire, and arrange backup care is essential to his success in college and/or the work world. Your child's relationship with his PCA requires a certain amount of emotional distance (your child is the employer/boss, the PCA is the employee) but can feel quite close in terms of the intimate personal care the PCA provides. While having a respectful relationship with one's PCA is a good thing, your child needs to be aware that problems will result if their roles become blurred by romantic or sexual entanglements, or if he and the PCA become too emotionally involved in each other's lives.

### Vocational Training and Employment

Not all kids who have disabilities go to college; some will transition to the work world right after high school. And many who do go to college

☛ A listing of every state's vocational department can be found on the U.S. Government Department of Education website: www.workworld.org/wwwebhelp/state_vocational_rehabilitation_vr_agencies.htm.

will need assistance finding a job afterward. There are several sources for vocational training and job placement that may be helpful for kids with either a high school or a college diploma.

Each state in the United States has a department of vocational rehabilitation (sometimes called "vocational services") whose mission is to help people who have disabilities become employed.

Any adult who has a disability is eligible for services. Benefits vary but may include evaluation of work skills and preferences, financial assistance with job training programs, partial payment of college tuition, assistance with job placement, and help negotiating accommodations with an employer.

Private, fee-for-service vocational rehabilitation and/or employment agencies and those located in freestanding rehabilitation centers, faith-based family service agencies, and nonprofit community agencies (such as Goodwill Industries) may also be helpful. If your child is enrolled at a college, the office on disability may provide career or job counseling and a job bank or list.

In addition to helping your child gain access to these vocational services, you can help prepare your child for working life by discussing a variety of career options. Your child who has a physical disability should be encouraged to follow his dreams, but you can also help her find a match between her interests and goals on the one hand and her abilities and disabilities on the other. Donny's parents, for instance, want him to

☛ Your child may also be eligible for vocational services through your state's Department of Developmental Disabilities. A listing for each state is available through the federal Administration on Developmental Disabilities: www.acf.hhs.gov/programs/add/state.html. Although the term "developmental disability" is often used to mean a disability that impairs cognitive function, it can also refer to any disability that begins before the age of 21.

know that there are "many choices he will have in life." But they tend to praise Donny for his intellectual abilities and social skills and have encouraged him to think about a career that relies on "brain power," like teaching. Donny is fascinated with engines and, like many boys, would like to be a mechanic or work on race cars. His parents support this interest but have suggested that he think about becoming an engineer or automotive designer, since his ability to use his hands is limited.

Susan, a young woman who has paraplegia, says she was interested in becoming a large animal veterinarian before her injury. After her injury, she rethought her options. She wanted to do something interesting and make a good income, "knowing I'd always have to work sitting down," so she "picked a practical major" (information technology) in college.

Teaching your children about disability laws, especially the Americans with Disabilities Act (ADA), can help them understand and take advantage of their legal rights in the areas of employment (the ADA also addresses access to public services and transportation). The ADA was signed into law in 1990, but its application continues to evolve based on new legal challenges. It provides protection against discrimination in hiring based on disability status and mandates that employers make reasonable accommodations for an employee who has a disability, as long as he can do the basic functions of his job. As a young adult applying for her first job, it's particularly important to know how to avoid discrimination in employment, beginning with the first interview. While employers may ask whether she can do the basic functions of the job (for example, can she use a computer for word processing), asking questions about your daughter's health or disability status is not allowed during the interview stage. Once offered the job, your son or daughter can decide whether to request accommodations (for example, a voice activation program or modified keyboard for the computer). There is no requirement to divulge any more information about one's health than is necessary to justify the request for these accommodations. Keeping abreast of the current interpretations of the ADA and other disability laws can add to your child's success in the work world (see the Resources section for the ADA website).

### Managing Medical and Physical Care

Scott, whose stepdaughter Celeste has OI, wants her to enjoy the independence of driving a car but worries about "who gets to her after a crash. Will the paramedics know how to treat a woman with OI?" Similarly, when he thinks of her going to college and living independently, he anticipates "no problems when she is healthy" but worries that if she has a bone break, she may not be able to fend for herself. While he thinks that a PCA might solve the problem, he still hopes she'll go to college close to home, so he and his wife can be her "emergency backup plan." His wife, Evelyn, on the other hand, is less concerned and thinks Celeste can go to college wherever she wants.

As they get older, giving your children some basic education about common health problems and gradually allowing them to have more input on medical and treatment decisions will help them learn how their bodies work, develop their own values and preferences regarding medical care, and ultimately take over responsibility for their own health management.

Jon, an adult with OI, says, "I appreciate that my family included me in treatment decisions, that they were straightforward and honest. That built trust. Parents should let kids be a large part of the decision-making team."

By the time *any* child goes to college or leaves home for a job, he should know how to take care of minor health problems himself and when to seek professional care. Every young adult should be able to recognize symptoms of strep throat, allergic reaction, and common viral infection; clean and dress a cut or scrape; be aware of situations that need emergency medical attention; know which over-the-counter medicines to take for minor illnesses; and so forth. Young people should also know about how to prevent illness—through regular exercise, weight control, moderate alcohol use, and safe sex. In addition to these basics, children who have physical disabilities need information specific to their physical or medical conditions; they have a right to be told the truth about their disability and will benefit from understanding the full range of medical and rehabilitation options available to them.

Ken's family began asking his opinions about his medical treatment when he was in elementary school. Although they made the ultimate decisions then, it was clear to Ken that his input and preferences were valued and taken into consideration. When Ken was in high school, the doctor proposed an operation that would have taken him out of school for half of his senior year. The family convened to look at all the pros and cons of the operation and considered its impact on Ken's life. They left the final decision up to Ken, figuring that he was old enough to make decisions about his own body. Ken didn't think the time away from friends and school was a good trade-off, since the potential improvement offered by the operation was small and there were some substantial risks. So he opted against it.

As part of the transition to adulthood, teens who have disabilities should become knowledgeable and responsible about their own health issues, developing a collaborative relationship with their health care providers. As parents, you played a role as a partner in your child's health care team; now it is up to your child to become part of the team herself. Teens can be encouraged to do things such as ordering their own catheter supplies, refilling medications, and scheduling their own medical appointments. Even before the teen years, all children can be given some responsibility for health behaviors (like doing exercises) and taught to do some of their own medical care (for example, using a glucometer to monitor blood sugar or taking regular medications independently). In fact, when kids establish a good routine of self-care before the teen years, they may be less likely to use neglect of their self-care as a means of rebellion against parents.

Connie, an able-bodied 21-year-old, was on a cycling trip miles from home when she suddenly came down with a severe sore throat. "I remembered my mom telling me how strep throat can go 'dormant' and later you can get kidney problems. I sort of heard her voice in my head saying, 'Get checked!' So I went to a local clinic right away. And it was a good thing, because I needed antibiotics."

Connie had both the information about the dangers of sore throat and the skills to find a health care clinic in an unfamiliar city. She did not need to call home for help, because she had been adequately coached by her mother in the past and knew what to do.

When your child has a physical disability, she will need to know all of these things—and more. Understanding his unique medical or physical vulnerabilities and knowing how to care for routine physical problems are essential. Celeste, for example, will need to learn how to manage her OI while she is away from home, especially what to do if she breaks a bone. On her own, or with her parents' input, she can create a plan that might include which doctor or hospital to call, when to call an ambulance, where she will recuperate, and how she will complete school assignments during her recovery. Celeste could carry an emergency information card with her at all times, giving basic information about OI, a website address for more information, the phone number for her primary doctor, and some basic steps for how to treat her in an emergency like a car crash. Most importantly, Celeste's knowledge of her physical and medical care needs should be so complete that she can explain to any health care provider what she needs.

Taking care of medical equipment is also important—for example, regularly cleaning a continuous positive airway pressure (CPAP) device or other respiratory machine, checking wheelchairs for loose screws or deflated tires, keeping the battery charged on an electric scooter, or checking for worn-down crutch tips. Once away from home, a young adult will need to be familiar with companies that service his special equipment and can supply backups while his equipment is being repaired.

### Sexuality, Dating, and Marriage

Donny, a 13-year-old who has a muscle disorder, just went to his first boy-girl party. He wants to get married and become a dad someday. Priscilla wondered whether her son Jason, who has spina bifida, would get a date for his senior prom. Sean hopes his daughter, a college senior who has CP, will find a marriage partner to share her life with. And Elsie is "concerned about my grandson finding someone to love him and to have a family."

Sexuality, dating, and marriage are essential aspects of adulthood. Most parents look forward to the day when their son or daughter gets married and starts a family. Parents want their child to have the fulfillment and security of a loving partnership—and they want to become grandparents!

But kids who have physical disabilities often face barriers to dating, sexual intimacy, and finding a marriage partner. They are bombarded with media images of physical "perfection" and may feel—even more than able-bodied kids, who also struggle to fit in—that they are unattractive or unlovable. As a parent, your acceptance of your child as a sexual being and your expectation that he will find a mate are essential in counteracting social stereotypes. You can help your child feel that she is lovable and has the qualities and abilities to be a good and competent partner or spouse.

Teens who have physical disabilities may have fewer opportunities for sexual "play" or experimentation than able-bodied kids and teens, and the standard sex education curriculum does not address all of their particular needs and concerns. Though teenagers who have disabilities have the same risks as other teens for getting a sexually transmitted disease or having an unplanned pregnancy, their ability to use the usual methods of prevention may be limited, requiring special education and coaching. Teens who have disabilities, especially girls, are also vulnerable to sexual exploitation and need to be taught to recognize and avoid sexual manipulation or abuse.

You can help promote your child's sexual health by filling in the gaps in her sex education, preferably before she becomes sexually active. Many parents talk with their kids about the "birds and the bees" before they reach puberty, as part of preparing them for the physical and emotional changes they will soon experience. Immunization against the sexually transmitted diseases hepatitis B and human papillomavirus are given routinely to boys and girls in middle school; these vaccinations can be springboards to conversations with your child about sexuality and dating.

Beyond the basics of safe sex and birth control, it's important to convey the information and values about love and relationships that you feel are essential, to share your hope that your child will one day have a loving relationship or marriage, and to educate your child (or help him find resources for education) about any sexual health or sexual function issues related to his particular disability.

Listen to your child's point of view, try to understand the attitudinal and physical barriers that make dating difficult for your child, and work with him to find solutions. This is another place where adult role models—individuals who have physical disabilities who are in intimate relationships, are married, and have children—can be helpful to your child.

Alma was dating Lenny, and they were thinking about marriage and children. Alma worried about how she would care for babies because she used crutches and braces. She remembered meeting Lauren, another young woman who walked with crutches, at a conference the previous year. She had heard from mutual friends that Lauren had recently had a baby. So Alma asked Lauren if she could visit her; she hoped to see how Lauren managed to care for her baby. Alma saw that Lauren had a lower, side-opening crib, allowing her to sit down to care for the baby. She could easily transfer him to a stroller, which she pushed around the house with her abdomen. Lauren was a happy and confident new mom. This visit gave Alma the confidence that she could manage being a mother, too. A few weeks after the visit, Alma and Lenny got engaged.

"When I'm 29, I want to be working as an engineer, be a professional hand cyclist, and be married—possibly with children."
—Lance, a young man with paraplegia

## The Next Step (for Mom and Dad)

Now that your kids are embarking on their own lives, you can take a moment to savor their incredible accomplishments—and your own! As your child who has a disability becomes an adult—not fully formed, but with definite personality characteristics and more mature ideas—you may be amazed by all that he *can* do. But as you did when you first found out that your child had a disability, you will once again have to reconcile the ideal with the real, let go of some old dreams, and celebrate the reality of your young adult child, with all his strengths and challenges.

In the next chapter, we explore this letting go—how parents move on from full-time parenting and gradually shift the focus from their children to themselves. Parents reflect on the personal growth they've experienced in the process of raising children, as well as the new process of building a life for themselves that goes beyond parenting.

**The O'Briens:** Parents working together to help their daughters develop individual talents, support one another, and practice their faith

Leigh and Sean met in college; they married right after Leigh's graduation and Sean started his military career. Leigh got pregnant sooner than expected. It was a difficult time for her; she missed going skiing or having a drink with Sean at the officers' club. It was a "downer" to have so little time as a young couple without kids, yet they were excited about starting a family. Because Sean's career involved frequent travel, they agreed that Leigh would be a stay-at-home mom.

Their daughter Eliza was born prematurely at twenty-eight weeks. Sean "didn't expect the severity of what was to follow": at two days of age, Eliza had a brain hemorrhage. Sean remembers their two-and-a-half-pound baby wearing an oxygen mask; the "good news" was that she didn't need a breathing tube. Leigh remembers that "all the other mothers were moved off the maternity ward with their babies; I was not."

Eliza stayed in the hospital for a month after the hemorrhage. Doctors said that the hemorrhage would cause motor skill problems, but no specific diagnosis was given. At first Sean demanded to have all the information, but a nurse in the neonatal unit cautioned him, "You don't want to know too much." She encouraged him to let things be revealed when it was timely. That helped Sean stop dwelling on the unknowns.

Leigh's mother traveled to see them, and they assumed she would be helpful because of her experience with Leigh's brother, who had Down syndrome. But when she heard about the brain hemorrhage, she became faint. She told them, "I can't believe this is happening to *me* again." Seeing that Leigh's mother could not be helpful to them, Sean put her on a return flight. "The baggage you have either helps or hurts you," he says. Sean's older brother also had a cognitive disability, and although his family was not able to give them "hands-on" help, they were emotionally supportive to him and Leigh.

Leigh began to notice physical differences between Eliza and other babies her age, including an inability to sit up unsupported. When she was 9 months old, with Sean recently deployed overseas, Leigh took Eliza for her first physical therapy evaluation and came home with a diagnosis: cerebral palsy (CP). She remains grateful to the therapist for her honesty and remembers that it was "nice to know what it was . . . but shocking to hear it without Sean there." Sean heard the news from Leigh on a long-distance phone call; he, too, had to cope with his feelings alone.

When Sean returned home, he became actively involved with Eliza's care. He experienced his own confrontations with the medical system, finding both "saints and morons in clinical garb." After watching Eliza go through a number of operations and uncomfortable procedures, Sean learned to make his own judgments of what would be helpful to his daughter. "I always ask myself, 'Does she really need this?'" He wonders if clinicians have to numb themselves to the impact of the treatments they administer, and he respects those who remain truly caring and humane toward the children they treat.

Leigh recalls a couple of bad experiences at the hospital. There was a resident who failed to check medicines when Eliza was in pain, and an inept technician who tried to insert an IV four times—until Leigh banned her from the hospital room. But in general, Leigh experienced the medical system as supportive and helpful. When she took Eliza for therapies, she was often told, "You are so lucky to have this little girl, bright and alert." She felt that, too.

Leigh and Sean were nervous about having another child, but Eliza was very social and they wanted her to be surrounded by siblings. They were five months pregnant with their second child when Sean was deployed to combat duty. Leigh sent him photos of 2½-year-old Eliza, driving her electric wheelchair around the house, occasionally bumping into walls and furniture.

Michelle was born while Sean was overseas. She was a quiet child. "I was more scared than willing to talk to strangers." As a little girl, she had few close friends but was part of the neighborhood group. She often mediated their disputes because she was sensitive and didn't like to see people get upset.

In the first grade Michelle first recognized that her sister had a disability. Eliza attended an accessible school outside the neighborhood. For convenience, Michelle went there, too, riding the bus with children who had disabilities. She found that the kids had good senses of humor, and she liked going with them. When Eliza started middle school, Michelle enrolled in the neighborhood elementary school.

Alice joined the sisterhood five years after Michelle. Self-motivated, she was always busy, into her own projects. Two years later, Sammi was born. Sean and Leigh had consistent expectations for all four girls: study hard, attend church services, participate in sports and music, and have dinner with the family every night.

Relationships with their parents are different for each sister. Eliza says her disability made it more difficult to connect with peers, and she feels lucky to have a close relationship with her mother, whom she considers her best friend. "I tell her most of what's going on. This is not a normal thing with my other friends." Still, there have been some "on and off" moments in their relationship. Leigh would like to see Eliza, now a college graduate, take more steps toward independence and stop procrastinating about getting a job. Eliza admits she's avoiding the job hunt, which she fears will be highly stressful.

Michelle and Alice are closer to their father. Michelle's role in the family parallels Sean's role in his, the second sibling in a family where the oldest had a disability. He and Michelle each felt they had to fill the role of the "oldest," taking on extra responsibility without, as Michelle says, "getting the glory of being first." She felt that her father wanted her to do the activities with him that required physical skill, such as woodworking, that he would have done with Eliza, if it were possible. Michelle says she's the one who takes the "heat" when there is any discord among the sisters.

Alice says, "Me and my dad are closer because we share sports and our games." Sean coached many of her teams over the years. "I took the blame for things the other players did. He talked with me about that; he said I would take the blame because he couldn't say those things to the other players." Although she understood Sean's rationale, sometimes it felt unfair.

The girls know that Leigh can easily get angry or sad, but that she quickly forgets about it. Having a stay-at-home mother is appreciated because she's there to listen or to take them shopping for shoes or "things for projects." They all admit that there are certain subjects they don't discuss with their mother—and that are shared just with friends.

The sisters have had their share of fights, but these lessened as they grew and the older ones moved on to college and beyond. The younger sisters credit their older siblings for listening to them and helping them with homework.

They are sensitive to each other's feelings. Eliza says, "If I weren't around, people would be able to go off and do things. They've never made me feel that way, I just know it." Michelle says that her sister's physical disability hasn't made a difference in their day-to-day lives, but it has kept them from sharing some experiences. "I always wanted to go skiing. Obviously Eliza's disability is the reason we didn't do it. But I don't want to hurt my sister." She also feels that because of Eliza, she is more sensitive to issues such as people illegally parking in disabled parking spots; "That bothers me," she admits.

Alice adds, "I do think about the way I talk, and what I say in front of Eliza and how it must make her feel, like 'Oh I hate to go to soccer practice.' Eliza says, 'At least you can play soccer.'" Alice advises siblings not to go places where their sibling who has a disability can't go. She also recommends helping younger children to deal with unusual situations affecting their sibling who has a disability. She recalls, for example, that her little sister, Sammi, "freaked out when Eliza had surgery and they put screws in her head."

Sean and Leigh tried assigning household jobs to each of the girls (for example, putting away their laundry); however, the girls often avoided doing their chores, and Sean admits they were terrible about enforcing it. He disagrees with Leigh about this area of parenting. Sean wants the girls to help more and is willing to reward them with an allowance. But Leigh thinks it's enough if the girls are good students and athletes and keep up their musical practice, so she asks Sean not to harangue them about chores. Alice agrees that chores are too stressful, added to the pressure to keep up her grades and do well in sports. But once Eliza and Michelle departed for college, Alice helped with the lawn mowing, and Sammi with dinner.

Leigh and Sean believed in promoting physical risks that made their daughters stronger. They allowed fewer risks in social activities. The daughters could go out only in groups until age 16; then they could date, but their parents controlled where they could go.

Sean says he has tried to do the same things with all four girls, and the sisters agree that their parents give them equal attention, and "no one person is favored." Eliza's disability influenced the choice of shared family activities but didn't prevent each girl from enjoying sports and recreation. Sean says, "We live our lives. We had a routine. We got Eliza out to watch her sisters in their sports, but then she did what she wanted to do, like horseback riding." He walked her on the horse, just as he coached the younger girls' teams.

As a teenager, Eliza had treatment for scoliosis, including halo traction (using a brace screwed into the skull); this felt so unfair to Leigh, after all Eliza had been through. Sometimes Leigh finds herself thinking about the imperfect world. "Why? Why you? Why her? Sometimes I feel angry." But then Leigh says, "We are more caring, and I attribute that to Eliza. Religion gives me hope and a reason for why things are the way they are. If I didn't have my faith I would see pain, hopelessness. Every life has meaning. You give something and you get something back." Although Sean has had some conflicts about his faith, he participates with Leigh in their religious community. "The tenets of my religion have helped. When you think of Christ's life, it was perfect. He truly lived by example. That brings you back to where you need to be. He was my philosophy teacher."

The daughters also find religion meaningful. Eliza still attends church weekly. "When I got mad because life hadn't worked out the way I wanted, I thought of good things that happened. So someone up there is watching. When I need help, I say a prayer." Michelle, now a college student, goes to church with her friends, sometimes more out of habit than belief, "but I feel guilty if I don't go." She relies on her faith during times of desperation. Alice, 13, and Sammi, 11, attend church with their parents and participate in religious education classes.

Sean appreciates the rewards of raising a family that includes a child who has a disability. He tells other fathers to accept their sons and daughters as individuals, not to let others' expectations about physical disability change the way you see your children, able-bodied or not. "Don't change them," says Sean. "Realize the gift of intellect. Our daughter who has a disability has bettered our family."

Leigh says that the experience of raising Eliza "has made me the person I am. I'm not shallow or self-absorbed. I have an appreciation of what she can't do and how well she handles it. Eliza's taught me." Sean agrees, saying, "Eliza made Leigh grow up. She began to stand up for herself and the children. It made her stronger, solid on her own two feet. I can't hold a candle to her."

By the same token, Leigh thinks that "parents have a right to enjoy themselves, to take needed breaks, to be who you are, not Eliza's or Melissa's, or Alice's or Sammi's mother." She does this by running and taking long walks. Now she's looking for a part-time job, after years of being a full-time mother.

When asked her perspective on mothering a "mixed bag" family, Leigh relates the story of raising a child who has a disability to planning a trip to Rome and ending up in Holland. "It's okay to wish you were in Rome, but you would miss the tulips and windmills of Holland. We have to accept where we are."

# 7

# Letting One Dream Go to Let Another Grow

--------------------------------------------------------------------

"Looking back, I wouldn't have changed a thing. Jason's disability made me a better person."

—LEE, A FATHER

"I'm more insightful, recognizing that life is not a bed of roses but it is still good. I'm thankful I'm alive."

—SUSIE, A MOTHER

"If you are selfish, when you have a child who has a disability, your self-centeredness will go out the window."

—MIA, A MOTHER

Life moves on and so do you! Once your children have left the nest, you begin a new phase of your journey, one in which the spotlight shifts from your children's lives to your own. Along the way, the dream of the *ideal* family has been discarded in favor of your *real* family. Your dreams for your children have been redefined, replaced by the ones *they've* dreamed for themselves—and are now making reality as they venture out into the world on their own. This is a transition point, a time to take stock, to envision what you want and to plan the next step forward in your own life. You let one dream go to let another grow, for both your children and yourself.

Swinging that spotlight from your children's lives to your own is both exciting and daunting. You may have a jumble of feelings, from sadness over the loss of your children from the nest (perhaps mixed with frustration about those who can't seem to fly away!), to pride in your children and happiness for them, to a sense of personal parental accomplishment.

For Priscilla, parenting was "the most important part of my life—

devoting time and effort to raise confident, well-educated, and happy individuals." She expected that both her children would go to college, and the whole family was overjoyed when son Jason, who has spina bifida, was admitted to a university far from home with a full scholarship. Priscilla was exhilarated by Jason's ability to move on with his life, relishing his success. "It's a huge accomplishment for him. It's normalcy, what every kids wants. He is able to do it!"

You may also feel some anxiety about how to pursue—or create—goals for your own life when responsibility for your children is no longer its chief focus. Deciding how to let your new dreams grow, using your talents and skills, is a journey to the unknown. It's filled with possibilities, but a little scary.

NOTE: Not all young adult children move out on their own entirely; some boomerang back home, especially in economically depressed times, when jobs are hard to find or may not pay enough to support an independent apartment, or when working full-time is impossible while pursuing an advanced degree. Some adult children have medical problems that bring them home, either because their parents can provide the best care or because they can't afford to hire private nurses or attendants. Dora and Ted's daughter is in her early thirties and has osteogenesis imperfecta (OI). Several times, after a medical situation requiring care, she moved into her parents' home until the problems resolved and then returned to her apartment. A key for parents in these situations is to treat returning adult children like adults—with both respect and expectations for grown-up behavior and responsibilities—and for their kids, in turn, to be respectful of their parents as people with their own lives.

If you live in a multigenerational family, you also need to have some boundaries for yourself, your grown children, and/or your parents, making sure everyone is clear about their responsibilities and that there is mutual respect for privacy. George and Elena share a home with their daughter and her family. Recently their young adult son Matt, who uses a wheelchair, returned home as he searched for a job. His parents told Matt that he would need to take his turn cooking and helping with upkeep of the house like everyone else in addition to taking care of his own personal needs. Expectations would be the same for all the adults in the family.

# Looking Back at What You've Learned

Raising a child who has a physical disability offers parents opportunities for personal growth. You are forced to rethink values, change priorities, and decide just how you want to spend your finite stores of time and energy. Having a child who has a disability leads parents to shuck old ideas of "normal" or "perfect" and redefine what is worthwhile and valuable.

While parents usually dwell on how their *children* react and adjust to life's challenges, you can also benefit from looking back on *your own* track record on life's roller coaster. You'll be surprised to see the many ways you've matured; for instance, Erica points out that she became less self-absorbed and shallow. The challenges of family life spur parents to grow and develop their capacity as human beings—to become more involved, patient, tolerant, or thankful for the "small things" in life.

Reviewing the character strengths and coping skills that helped you raise your family can embolden you, providing the confidence to move forward into the next phase of life.

## Confidence in Yourself

Being a parent to that mixed-bag family of able-bodied children and those who have physical disabilities, you've grown many capacities, including belief in yourself. This self-confidence developed—sometimes through trial and error—as you mastered the skills necessary to raise *all* your children and accumulated the unique knowledge and technical know-how to meet the needs of your child who has a physical disability. You've managed difficult medical and physical routines, learned the professional lingo, and made tough decisions.

In that process, you've collected a toolbox full of capabilities and "cope-abilities" to help you over the physical and emotional bumps in the road. Remember "going around the cone"—the first time an emergency or unexpected medical problem arose, and the exhaustion and self-doubt you went through? But each time you went around that "cone," you felt more confident in your ability to handle the situation because you survived the previous trip and had your own personal book of remedies. In coping with an array of problems and emergencies and—oh yes!—

triumphs, you developed your own patterns to guide you. These patterns became models for your children, too, showing them how to be proactive, to rely on experience as a guide, to be flexible in considering their options, and to act decisively in emergencies.

You've made decisions, created your own expectations of family life, adapted to unfamiliar medical and rehabilitation care routines, taken frequent detours (ramps in hidden places!), and met a slew of professionals (brace makers, surgeons, rehabilitation counselors) you never thought you'd need—all in a day's work! You are well prepared for your next steps into the world beyond parenting.

## Trusting Your Instincts

Like Kelsey, whose daughter has spina bifida, you developed more trust in your own inner voice or gut instinct as time progressed. "At one point we felt something just wasn't right with our daughter, and it turned out we were correct—she needed surgery." Often "gut instinct" reflects the deep personal knowledge you have of your child—which you may not be aware of on a conscious level and can't fully explain. You just *know*. By listening to your gut or inner voice, you learned to trust your judgment about your child's condition, to know when to get help.

"Gut checks" are important not only in decisions about your children but also in many other decision-making situations. Now you can apply this tool, along with others that have worked in the past, to decisions you make about yourself in this new, more "adult-centric" stage of life.

---

**T**We can judge our satisfaction with decisions we make with our brains by listening to our guts. Think back to a decision you made recently and how you felt in the pit of your stomach at the time. If you felt queasy or jittery inside, it may be because you weren't ready to make the decision owing to lack of information, or because you were making a decision for the wrong reasons—perhaps to please someone else or as a result of pressure from peers or a professional. But if your "insides" feel settled and calm after making a decision, it is probably the right one for you.

---

## Balancing Self-Sufficiency with Help from Others

Living life well requires balance. As a parent of multiple children, one of whom has a physical disability, you've had to build self-sufficiency, resilience, and confidence in your independent judgments. This had to be balanced by a certain amount of support from others. In the beginning, you might have been uncomfortable accepting help because you felt unworthy, didn't want to feel beholden to someone else, or were afraid of being a burden. But as you recognized your limits, you learned to ask for help, allowing yourself to rely on others when necessary. Mia, a single mother whose youngest child has OI, says, "At first I had to prove I could do everything. Now I can accept help. I rely on others. You have to build your support system so you are not all by yourself." Susie, whose twins have physical disabilities, became a gracious recipient of help when she realized that she could repay that help in the future by giving the gift of her time or presence to someone else in need. Pili found her help through a support group of parents with both able-bodied children and those who have physical disabilities. "It's incredible to share your journey with parents of kids who have other disabilities."

Balancing may also involve getting professional help, which is beneficial, even to expert parents, when they are feeling bogged down by life. Opening up to a mental health professional or parenting expert helps some parents get the breathing room to assess their options in a tough situation, often leading to better understanding of the issues and a change in how they handle the problem or cope with their emotions. Emma, a teacher and now a parent herself who has spina bifida, had parents who divorced when she was young. She wishes her parents had reached out to experts. "You can't meet the needs of your family if your head is not clear, if you don't have strategies. Dealing with professionals can be a huge support for overwhelmed parents."

Professional counseling can also be useful when you first find yourself in an empty nest and feel unsure of how to get on with your life. Valerie, the mother of five children, including a son who uses a wheelchair, was a stay-at-home parent who gave up her real estate business to care for her family. When her youngest daughter left for college, Valerie felt depressed, unanchored, and useless. After some weeks of tearfulness and withdrawal from her usual social schedule, her husband encouraged her to "go talk with someone." Once she examined her feelings of loss and abandonment with her therapist, Valerie was able to see that her children felt free to "fly solo" largely because of the good job she had done as a parent. She also came to understand that the skills she had given to her children were the same ones she herself could use in this next stage of life—in order to fly on her own or in tandem with her husband.

## Turning Anger into Action

You've found that the energy behind negative feelings can be used for positive results if harnessed creatively. As the parent of a child who has a physical disability, you know the frustration and anger you've felt when your child was excluded from activities, exposed to prejudice or teasing, or unable to get around barriers to play, socialize, or go to school with his peers. Although anger is usually seen as a "negative" emotion, its bound-up energy can actually be channeled into constructive action. Runner found that when he turned his anger into fuel for the fight to meet his child's medical and social needs, he was able to conquer his feelings of helplessness. An everyday "anger arouser" is the abuse of handicapped parking spaces by people who do *not* have a disability. Marian turned her ire into action by putting official-looking notices on the windshields of cars illegally parked in these spaces. It was a small constructive gesture, but she was taking action. She hoped it would make people think twice about what they were doing and perhaps change their illegal parking habits.

Some parents get angry and frustrated with the obstacles faced not only by their own children but by *all* kids who have disabilities. Their anger motivates them to advocate for better services, increase awareness, and support legislation that can improve the lives of all children. Regina, energized by her indignation at the fact that her child had no accessible entrance to the municipal pool, led a letter writing campaign to the town council, resulting in the installation of curb cuts and an accessible bathroom. Other parents have taken a similar route, writing to legislators requesting power-operated doors, accessible bus routes, special walkways into parks and recreational areas, and many other accommodations.

If you've raised a child who has a physical disability amid your brood, you may have a built-in radar screen for social justice and child welfare in general. Luke, whose teenage son was born prematurely, gets angry when other parents act without regard for the well-being of their kids, "for example, when I read an article about a pregnant woman using cocaine." Billy feels his "blood boil" when he sees parents yelling at or slapping their children. Once your own children are out on their own, you may contribute to the well-being of other children and their families, perhaps through organized political action or through one-on-one help.

## Increasing Patience and Tolerance

Hard-driving parents who felt stressed when they had to adjust their busy schedules to the slower timetables of children, especially those who have physical disabilities, found that their patience grew through parenting. In addition, the external demands of the medical or rehabilitation system required them to slow down and helped them develop the ability to wait, endure, and be steady. Veteran parents say they had to "pump up" their patience and learn greater tolerance.

As the father of four daughters, Sean often felt his patience tried—and worked at increasing it. He developed the awareness that every person has "trials and tribulations"; it's the way we deal with our circumstances that determines how they affect us. Sean was active in his daughters' lives, coaching soccer and joining in therapeutic horseback riding; he turned what others might perceive as a "trial" into a positive experience, learning to adjust his timetable to each daughter's different tempo and be tolerant of their varying needs.

Cindy also found greater tolerance and empathy for others through her experience as the mother of a child who has a physical disability. She accepts certain behaviors she formerly would not put up with, understanding that a person might just be having "a bad day." She knows that when people are dealing with events in their lives that are beyond their control they may not act in a civil manner. "I'm easier on others," she says.

Lee says that joining his son Jason in activities such as going to the rifle range in his wheelchair has made him "more understanding, patient, and flexible." Mary agrees; although parenting a child who has a physical disability involved more work and fatigue, she says that her patience and tolerance have grown and she has learned to reach out to others. "You grow with it or you grow bitter." Mary has learned to be more gentle and understanding not only with others but with herself as well.

Grandparents often go through positive changes that parallel your experience as parents. Elsie says that "having a grandchild who has a disability made a huge difference. It made us more patient and understanding of other people who also have something to carry." This understanding brought her greater tolerance for human diversity beyond her family. As she reached out to her community, Elsie's faith in people and hope for the future were bolstered by discovering how much other people cared for her grandson and their family.

## Looking Ahead to What You Want

When you find yourself in your new post-active-parenting status, you feel a bit rudderless, as if your focus is fuzzy. You may still be working outside the home, and there are likely to be some needs you continue to fill for your kids or other family members. Perhaps you remember a similar time as you transitioned from single to married or from being a couple to having children. But this phase of life has a different tone; you are a different person, intellectually and emotionally, as a result of your life experiences. Your interests, occupation, ideas, and belief systems have evolved, changed, or solidified over time.

One of the biggest challenges for parents at this stage is to define where they want to go, what they want to do. Do they want a sea change or to stay steady? Do you feel stumped by the question "What do I want out of life?" Are you sure of your dreams and how to reach them? Do you stay with familiar horizons or explore new ones?

Shifting away from 24/7 parenting allows you to put into effect the plans you've been waiting to execute, or to invest your energy in figuring out a new dream or goal. Whether your goals are clear or you are still searching, the next phase of life will likely bring something new in work or study, hobbies or interests, reconnecting with your spouse or partner, rebuilding your social life, taking care of yourself, or pursuing your passions. There is a world of possibilities ahead of you.

## Working and Studying

Do you want to devote more time to your career, or start a new one? If you were a stay-at-home mom or dad, decisions about returning to work can be perplexing. Do you return to what you did before having children or go in another direction? Runner, a stay-at-home dad and computer expert, found that by the time he was ready to go back to work, his skills were out of date in the fast-changing field of computer science. If you experience something similar, more education or skills training may be what you need. On the other hand, you may decide that your former job doesn't sound fulfilling or exciting anymore. Perhaps your interests have changed; maybe you were a nurse and no longer want to be a caregiver. Or, like Susie, whose twin boys had physical disabilities, you might choose to turn your knowledge of parenting and disability into professional advocacy work for other families in need of education and support. If you are financially and physically able, you might want to push the envelope even further—join the Peace Corps or do missionary work abroad or begin a non-profit group—or just retire! Leigh, with two kids in and two out of the home, prepared herself early for the empty nest to come by looking for part-time work, so she could gradually reorient herself to the workaday world, figure out what type of work she wanted to do, and be ready to take on a full-time job after all her daughters were living away from home.

## Hobbies and Interests

Parents who stay involved with their hobbies, athletics, arts, reading, and other interests during the children's growing-up years will be in a better position to make the transition from full-time parents to parents of young adults. They have their sources of enjoyment ready to fill the time that is freed when children are grown. Rather than feeling that time is weighing heavily on their hands after the kids leave, these parents report that they become so engaged in pursuing their interests that there just aren't enough hours in the day to do all they want. Priscilla, for instance, always nurtured herself with supportive friends, involvement in volunteer work, church activities, and scrapbooking, even while raising Jason and

Jean. Although still employed, she has time to become more deeply involved with these activities that she finds so satisfying.

## Reconnecting with Your Spouse or Partner

Perhaps in the turmoil of raising a family, you had little opportunity to talk to your cocaptain about your own relationship. You may have grown apart in your ideas and attitudes, or you may not have had the energy to be there for each other in difficult times. When your child was going through a medical crisis, you and your spouse became focused on his ordeal, at times leaving you without each other's emotional support. Later you talked about it and apologized to one another, working out ways to do better next time. Now you have time to put in the effort to reconnect and strengthen your bonds of trust and intimacy.

## Rebuilding Your Social Life

Now that you are less connected on a day-to-day basis with your children, you can focus on nurturing other relationships, not only with your partner, but also with family members and friends. You may be a single parent and want to find someone with whom to share your life. Some single parents have found others in the same boat at national disability group meetings. Other parents have joined faith-based adult groups, interest clubs, and athletic teams, as well as online dating services.

Friendships—old and new—can be more fully developed and savored. Now you have more time for dropping by a friend's home for coffee or going to a movie in the middle of the day or having a gossip session with friends on the front porch. You probably have friends who are "mine" and friends who are "ours"—those you like to have lunch with on your own and others whom you and your significant other enjoy together. Whether single or married, getting into the swing of things with other people breathes new energy into your life—mentally, emotionally, and physically. You can deepen your existing friendships or widen your social circle by talking about books with friends, analyzing movies you've seen together, learning to salsa dance, participating in political campaigns, organizing a gourmet dinner club, going on a weekend retreat, rooting for your favorite teams, teaming up to help build homes for those in need, or playing in a community band—the list of possibilities goes on.

## Taking Care of Yourself

Whether a single or co-parent, you may not have had much—or any—time to take care of yourself while on full-time parent duty. Now there may be extra time during the week or on weekends, formerly taken up by kid-oriented activities, in which you can think about your body's needs—exercise, diet, skin care, relaxation. Some parents are able to make this a priority even while raising kids; Evelyn's husband Scott always supported her so she could get plenty of rest and care for herself by exercising and eating right. But most parents have not been able to accomplish this when their time and energies were concentrated on their children's needs. It may feel strange at first to give yourself permission to work out at the gym, go for a run, or take a long walk. Some couples build an exercise program for two, going for long walks, jogging, swimming, playing tennis, or working out in the gym together. They find increased levels of energy and a general feeling of well-being. As one parent observed, "It helps sustain my sense of self." April and Runner, both avid physical fitness advocates, found that running, both together and solo, helped reduce the stress of the tough medical events they went through with son Lance. It is still an integral part of their lives.

## Pursuing Your Passions

You are fortunate if you have interests that are engrossing and engaging. But if you can go beyond that and find your *passion*, life is even better! Passion is a compelling desire to be involved in something you can "lose yourself" in. Have you ever felt like the world, with all its demands and questions, melted away? Maybe in the thick of a math problem, or working out the next line of a poem, or finding the right blue for the sky in your painting, you suddenly found that time had flown by. Your passion might be adding to your knowledge about the Mayan culture, learning to play *Rhapsody in Blue* on the piano, visiting all the state capitols, or compiling your family history. Exploring (or perhaps discovering) your passion keeps you developing and thriving when your children have left home. Jana, whose daughter has rheumatoid arthritis, found that, partly as a result of parenting experience, she was able to build her confidence as a sculptor and to pursue this passion after her daughter went to college. Jana applied the four elements she used to raise her resilient daughter to her own life—she took responsibility for her work ethic, experienced many aspects of her work, took risks on "beyond the realm" pieces, and expanded her social life by reaching out to others through her art.

### Giving Back

When Susie was a newly divorced young mother of four, her wise friend advised her to accept help because she could repay it by helping others later. Susie listened: she has helped link numerous people who have disabilities to the services they need and to each other. She channeled her professional expertise and her volunteer energy into her passion, giving back what she was given tenfold.

Giving back is a fulfilling aspect of many parents' lives. A kind word or gesture that shows understanding for those in the same boat, especially young families, is a simple way to help others.

Many parents, like the Fishers, make fund-raising a key component of their giving back. The whole family is involved in fund-raisers, including Grandmother Ann, who solicits "goodies" to make baskets that are auctioned to raise money for the OI Foundation. D. K. actively solicits contributions from big corporations to fund research on OI.

## Moving Forward

You've been gifted with both able-bodied children and those who have physical disabilities. You've discovered that children are children, but the child who has a physical disability has extra unknowns to deal with. You've raised your kids, coped with ups and downs and medical "surprises," made sure each child was included, instilled in them your knowledge, helped them develop their own value system, prepared them with competencies, created fun times for them, laughed with and listened to them, and finally helped them out of the nest—in short, you have cared well for your gifts. You've discovered what inclusive parenting is all about. Now it's time to direct that caring energy toward yourself, to grow the dreams that will fulfill your potential and increase your resiliency as you move forward with your life.

Remember that, as you go about the business of life after parenting, you are still a role model for your adult children—just as you were a model for parenting when you raised them. You will continue to create new patterns of living that your children can learn from and emulate—if they choose. And wouldn't it be wonderful if, when your kids reach the empty nest stage themselves, they remember the joy and gusto with which you embraced it?

# Resources

----------------------------------------------------------------------------

## Accessibility

*Accessible Home Design: Architectural Solutions for the Wheelchair User*, 2nd ed.
Published by Paralyzed Veterans of America
801 Eighteenth Street NW
Washington, DC 20006-3517

Amherst Homes, Inc.
7378 Charter Cup Lane
Westchester, OH 45069
Phone: 513-891-3303

The Center for Universal Design
North Carolina State University, Box 8613
Raleigh, NC 27695-8613
Phone: 800-647-6777
www.design.ncsu.edu

Concrete Change
600 Dancing Fox Road
Decatur, GA 30032
Phone: 404-378-7455
www.concretechange.org
Mission is to make every home "visitable."

Lifease, Inc.
2451 Fifteenth Street NW
New Brighton, MN 55112
Phone: 612-636-6869
www.lifease.com

United States Access Board
www.access-board.gov
An independent federal agency whose primary mission is technical assistance on accessibility for people who have disabilities.

## Accessible Transportation and Travel

Access-Able Travel Source
PO Box 1796
Wheat Ridge, CO 80034
www.access-able.com

Accessible Europe
Phone: 011-39-011-30-1888
www.accessibleurope.com
Travel agencies specializing in accessible tours and travel in Europe and beyond.

Accessible Journeys
Phone: 800-846-4537
www.disabilitytravel.com
Organizes wheelchair travel for groups and individuals, including cruises.

*The Air Carrier Access Act: Make It Work for You*
Published by Paralyzed Veterans of America
801 Eighteenth Street NW
Washington, DC 20006-3517

Emerging Horizons
www.emerginghorizons.com
Accessible travel news and information
for travelers who have disabilities.

International Association for Medical
Assistance to Travelers
Phone: 716-754-4883
www.iamat.org
Provides access to English-speaking
medical care providers for English
speakers traveling in foreign countries.

*New Horizons: Information for the Air
Traveler with a Disability*
United States Department of
Transportation
Aviation Consumer Protection Division,
C-75
400 Seventh Street, SW
Washington, DC 20590
http://airconsumer.ost.dot.gov/
publications/horizons.htm
The website has the full text of the
document.

Society for Accessible Travel and
Hospitality
www.sath.org
A nonprofit organization for travelers
who have disabilities.

Travelin' Talk Network
www.travelintalk.net
A network of over one thousand people
who offer help and services to
travelers who have disabilities.
Membership benefits include discounts
at various motels.

### Assistance Dogs

Assistance Dogs International, Inc.
www.assistancedogsinternational.org/
assistancedogproviders.php
Accredits guide dog programs involved
in training either service or hearing
dogs.

### Becoming a Parent When You Have a Physical Disability

http://raisingchildren.net.au/articles/
parents_with_physical_disability.html
Australian parenting site with stories of
parents who have physical disabilities
and have raised families.

www.lookingglass.org
Organization focusing on parents or
children who have disabilities which
provides training, does research, and
disseminates information.

### Books and Magazines for Teens Who Have a Physical Disability

Cheney, Glenn Ann. *Teens with Physical
Disabilities: Real-Life Stories of
Meeting the Challenges.* Springfield,
NJ: Enslow, 1995.

Kriegsman, Kay H., Zaslow, Elinor L.,
and D'Zmura-Rechsteiner, Jennifer.
*Taking Charge: Teenagers Talk about
Life and Physical Disabilities.*
Bethesda, MD: Woodbine House,
1992.

New Horizons Un-Limited Inc.
www.new-horizons.org/libmag.html
Lists magazines and periodicals for
people who have disabilities.

Stewart, Gail B. *Teens with Disabilities.*
San Diego, CA: Lucent Books, 2001.

Thornton, Denise. *Physical Disabilities:
It Happened to Me: The Ultimate
Teen Guide.* Lanham, MD: Scarecrow,
2007.

### Books for Children Who Have a Physical Disability

Carter, Alden R., and Carter, Carol S.
*Stretching Ourselves: Kids with
Cerebral Palsy.* Park Ridge, IL: Albert
Whitman, 2000.

Dobbs, Jean. *Kids on Wheels—A Young Person's Guide to Wheelchair Lifestyle*. Horsham, PA: No Limits Communications, 2004.

Heelan, Jamee R., and Simmonds, Nicola. *Rolling Along: The Story of Taylor and His Wheelchair*. Chicago: Rehabilitation Institute of Chicago Learning Books, 2000.

Lutkenhoff, Marlene, and Oppenheim, Sonya, eds. *SPINAbilities: a Young Person's Guide to Spina Bifida*. Bethesda, MD: Woodbine House, 1997.

### College Resources
Disability Friendly Colleges
www.disabilityfriendlycolleges.com

"Finding the Right College Fit for Students with Physical Disabilities"
www.klemmerec.com/resources
_reading_article_disabilities.htm

HEATH Resource Center
www.heath.gwu.edu
A national clearinghouse on post-secondary education for individuals who have disabilities.

### Dating, Sexuality, and Marriage
American Association of Sexuality Educators, Counselors, and Therapists
PO Box 1960
Ashland, VA 23005-1960
Phone: 804-752-0026
www.aasect.org

American Society for Reproductive Medicine
1209 Montgomery Highway
Birmingham, AL 35216-2809
Phone: 205-978-5000
www.asrm.org

Ducharme, Stanley H., and Gill, Kathleen M. *Sexuality after Spinal Cord Injury: Answers to Your Questions*. Baltimore: Paul Brookes, 1997.

A Guide and Resource Directory to Male Fertility following SCI/C: A Miami Project Resource. www.themiami project.org

Kaufman, Miriam, Silverberg, Cory, and Odette, Fran. *The Ultimate Guide to Sex and Disability: For All of Us Who Live with Disabilities, Chronic Pain and Illness*. San Francisco: Cleis, 2003.

Rogers, Judith. *The Disabled Woman's Guide to Pregnancy and Birth*. New York: Demos Medical, 2006.

### Diagnosis-Specific Books and Resources
Determined 2 Heal
8112 River Falls Drive
Potomac, MD 20854
Phone: 703-795-5711
www.determined2heal.org
Information on psychosocial recovery, support, research, and prevention of SCI.

Dollar, Ellen Painter. *Growing Up with OI: A Guide for Families and Caregivers*. Tampa, FL: Osteogenesis Imperfecta Foundation, 2001.

Hill Foundation
737 N. Michigan Avenue
Suite 1560
Chicago, IL 60611
Phone: 312-284-2525
www.facingdisability.com
A website that provides information about families living with spinal cord injury, as well as peer role modeling, support, and peer counseling.

Lutkenhoff, Marlene, ed. *Children with Spina Bifida: A Parents' Guide.* Bethesda, MD: Woodbine House, 1999.

Palmer, Sara, Kriegsman, Kay H., and Palmer, Jeffrey B. *Spinal Cord Injury: A Guide for Living*, 2nd ed. Baltimore: Johns Hopkins University Press, 2008.

Thompson, Charlotte. *Raising a Child with a Neuromuscular Disorder.* New York: Oxford University Press, 1999.

### Disability Rights
Americans with Disabilities Act (ADA) Information
Phone: 800-466-4ADA
www.ada.gov

Disability Rights Education and Defense Fund (DREDF)
2212 Sixth Street
Berkeley, CA 94710
Phone: 415-644-2555
Provides information on disability rights laws and policy. Publishes a free newsletter, *Disability Rights News.*

### Driving and Vehicle Adaptation
*Adapting Motor Vehicles for People with Disabilities*
www.nhtsa.gov/cars/rules/adaptive/brochure/brochure.html
A brochure published by the National Highway Traffic Safety Administration.

*Adaptive Automotive Equipment: A Consumer's Guide*
www.unitedspinal.org/pdf/ahc.pdf
A brochure published by the United Spinal Association.

Association for Driver Rehabilitation Specialists (ADED)
PO Box 49
Edgerton, WI 53534
Phone: 608-884-8833
www.driver-ed.org; www.aded.net

Family Village
www.familyvillage.wisc.edu/at/driving.htm
Adaptive driving and vehicle adaptation sources.

### Equipment and Technology
Abledata
8455 Colesville Road, Suite 935
Silver Spring, MD 20910
Phone: 800-227-0216
www.abledata.com
Maintains a database with over 15,000 listings of adaptive devices for all disabilities.

Assistive Technology News
www.atechnews.com
Featuring articles on new assistive technologies for people who have disabilities.

Karp, Gary. *Choosing a Wheelchair: A Guide for Optimal Independence.* Sebastopol, CA: O'Reilly and Associates, 1998.

Sammons Preston and Enrichments
PO Box 5071
Bolingbrook, IL 60440-5071
Phone: 800-323-5547;
fax: 800-547-4333
A mail-order catalog for accessibility aids.

### Grandparents Raising Grandchildren

AARP Grandparent Information Center
www.aarp.org/relationships/friends -family/grandfacts-sheets
Information and links to a variety of resources for grandparents. Includes fact sheets that list resources in each state in the country.

Grandparenting Today
www.uwex.edu/ces/flp/grandparent/
Run by the University of Wisconsin Extension Service, this website offers links to national resources and publication. Includes a listing of books about grandparents raising grand-children at http://learningstore.uwex .edu/assets/pdfs/B3786-9.pdf.

www.grandparents.com
Offers information and links to a variety of resources for grandparents.

### Housing Assistance for People Who Have Disabilities

*Fair Housing: How to Make the Law Work for You*
Washington, DC
Available electronically from Paralyzed Veterans of America at www.pva.org.

United States Department of Housing and Urban Development
Office of Fair Housing and Equal Opportunity
451 Seventh Street, SW
Washington, DC 20410
Phone: 202-708-1112
www.hud.gov
Provides information on housing rights and resources for people who have disabilities and for those who encounter discrimination in housing.

### Medicaid Information

Centers for Medicare and Medicaid Services (CMS)
United States Department of Health and Human Services
www.cms.hhs.gov
Information on Medicare and Medicaid benefits and programs, the Medicaid Waiver, and other programs and services provided by these government health insurance programs.

### National Mental Health Organizations

American Association of Marriage and Family Therapists
112 South Alfred Street
Alexandria, VA 22314-3061
Phone: 703-838-9808

American Psychiatric Association
1000 Wilson Boulevard, Suite 1825
Arlington, VA 22209
Phone: 800-35-PSYCH
www.psych.org

American Psychological Association
750 First Street, NE
Washington, DC 20002
Phone: 800-374-2721
www.apa.org

National Association of Social Workers
750 First Street, NE, Suite 700
Washington, DC 20002
Phone: 202-408-8600
www.socialworkers.org

### Organizations and Foundations
Amputee Coalition of America
900 East Hill Avenue, Suite 290
Knoxville, TN 37915
Phone: 888-267-5669
www.amputee-coalition.org

Arthritis Foundation
PO Box 7669
Atlanta, GA 30357
Phone: 800-283-7800
www.arthritis.org

Muscular Dystrophy Association (USA)
3300 East Sunrise Drive
Tucson, AZ 85718
Phone: 800-572-1717
www.mdausa.org

National Organization for Rare
  Disorders
55 Kenosia Avenue
Danbury, CT 06810
Phone: 800-999-6673
www.rarediseases.org

National Spinal Cord Injury
  Association
75-20 Astoria Boulevard
Jackson Heights, NY 11370
Phone: 718-803-3782
www.spinalcord.org

National Stroke Association
9707 East Easter Lane, Suite B
Centennial, CO 80112
Phone: 800-787-6537
www.stroke.org

Osteogenesis Imperfecta Foundation
804 West Diamond Avenue, Suite 210
Gaithersburg, MD 20878
Phone: 301-947-0083
www.oif.org

Spina Bifida Association
4590 McArthur Boulevard NW,
  Suite 250
Washington, DC 20007
Phone: 800-621-3141
www.spinabifidaassociation.org

United Cerebral Palsy
1825 K Street NW, Suite 600
Washington, DC 20006
Phone: 800-872-5827
www.ucp.org

www.disaboom.com
Website with links to a variety of
  disability organizations.

### Parenting a Child Who Has a Physical Disability
Albrecht, Donna. *Raising a Child Who Has a Physical Disability*. New York: John Wiley and Sons, 1995.

Balshaw, Mark L. *When Your Child Has a Disability*. Baltimore: Paul H. Brookes, 2001.

Brooks, Robert, and Goldstein, Sam. *Raising Resilient Children*. New York: McGraw-Hill, 2011.

Children and Physical Disabilities
www.findingdulcinea.com/guides/Health/Physical-Disabilities.pg_02.html
Provides information dealing with all aspects of physical disability, as well as resources for sports, activities, socialization, camps, etc.

National Dissemination Center for Children with Disabilities
www.nichcy.org
A central source of information on disabilities in children of all ages. Includes easy-to-read information on IDEA, the law authorizing early intervention services and special education. State Resource Sheets help you connect with disability agencies and organizations in your state.

www.fathersnetwork.org
Resources for fathers of children with special needs.

### Sports, Recreation, and Camping

Active Living Magazine: Adapted Activities, Products and Places
Disability Today Publishing Group, Inc.
PO Box 2660, Niagara Falls, NY 14302
www.activelivingmagazine.com

Adaptive Outdoorsman
www.adaptiveoutdoorsman.com/handicaphunting
A website for hunters who have disabilities.

American Canoe Association
7432 Alban Station Boulevard, Suite B-226
Springfield, VA 22159-2311

Buckmasters American Deer Foundation
www.badf.org

Handicapped Scuba Association International
1104 El Prado
San Clemente, CA 92672-4637
Independent scuba diver training and certifying agency. Offers Dive Buddy Program.

International Paralympic Committee
www.paralympic.org

Mersey River Chalets
Nova Scotia, Canada
www.merseyriverchalets.ns.ca
Accessible accommodations and nature activities.

*Murderball* (film, available on DVD and video). Codirected by Henry Alex Rubin and Dana Adam Shapiro. Produced by Jeffrey Mandell and Dana Alex Shapiro. Documentary about wheelchair rugby and the journey of the American "quad" rugby team to the Paralympics. (See also United States Quad Rugby Association, below.)

National Ability Center
Park City, UT
Phone: 435-694-3991
www.discovernac.org
Specializes in accessible recreation, sports, and leisure activities.

National Association of Handicapped Outdoor Sportsmen, Inc.
RR 6, Box 25, Centralia, IL 62801

National Center on Physical Activity and Disability
Phone: 800-900-8086
www.ncpad.org

National Foundation of Wheelchair Tennis
940 Calle Amanecer, Suite B
San Clemente, CA 92672

National Wheelchair Basketball
  Association
110 Seaton Building
University of Kentucky
Lexington, KY 40506
www.nwba.org

North American Riding for the
  Handicapped Association, Inc.
  (NARHA)
PO Box 33150
Denver, CO 80238
www.narha.org

Rocky Mountain Village
PO Box 115
Empire, CO 80438
www.eastersealsco.org

United States Golf Association
PO Box 708
Far Hills, NJ 07931
Modified rules for golfers who have
  disabilities.

United States Handcycling Federation
PO Box 2245
Evergreen, CO 80437

United States Paralympians Association
  (part of the United States Olympic
  organization) www.teamUSA.org/
  US-Paralympics.aspx
The Paralympics provides appropriate
  levels of competition within sports
  categories for athletes who have
  various types of disability.

United States Quad Rugby Association
5821 White Cypress Drive
Lake Worth, FL 22467-6230
www.quadrugby.com

Wheelchair Sports USA
10 Lake Circle, Suite G19
Colorado Springs, CO 80906
Information on archery, shooting,
  swimming, table tennis, weight lifting,
  track and field, and specifics on local
  competition.

Wilderness Inquiry, Inc.
1313 Fifth Street, PO Box 84
Minneapolis, MN 55414
Phone: 800-728-0719
www.wildernessinquiry.org
Land and water wilderness excursions
  for both able-bodied people and those
  who have disabilities.

Wilderness on Wheels Foundation
7125 West Jefferson Avenue, #155
Lakewood, CO 80235
Accessible camping, hiking, and fishing.

www.kidscamps.com/special_needs/
  physical_disability.html
Lists of camps for kids who have
  physical disabilities (can filter by
  region, age, length of stay, or camp
  type).

### Support for Siblings
Sibling Support Project
A Kindering Center Program
6512 23rd Avenue NW, #213
Seattle, WA 98117
www.siblingsupport.org
Sibshops and other resources for siblings
  of a child who has a disability.

### Visual and Performing Arts
Encore Studio for the Performing Arts
www.encorestudio.org
A professional theater company for
  people who have disabilities.

Mouth and Foot Painting Artists
2070 Peachtree Court, Suite 101
Atlanta, GA 30341
Phone: 770-986-7764
www.mfpausa.com

National Arts and Disability Center
www.semel.ucla.edu/nadc
Working for full inclusion of artists and
audiences with disabilities in the arts
community.

That Uppity Theater Company
4466 West Pine Boulevard, Suite 13C
St. Louis, MO 63108
Phone: 314-995-4600
www.uppityco.com
A theater company for both able-bodied
actors and those who have disabilities.

VSA Arts
818 Connecticut Avenue NW, Suite 600
Washington, DC 20006
Phone: 800-933-8721
www.vsarts.org
This nonprofit organization provides
opportunities for people who have
disabilities to learn through, participate in, and enjoy visual and
performing arts.

### Vocational Rehabilitation and Employment

State Vocational Rehabilitation
www.workworld.org/wwwebhelp/state
_vocational_rehabilitation_vr
_agencies.htm
Under the provisions of the Rehabilitation Act, every state government offers
vocational rehabilitation services to
help people who have disabilities
obtain education and job training and
return to gainful employment. A list of
state vocational rehabilitation agencies
can be found online.

United States Department of Labor's
Office of Disability Employment
Policies
www.dol.gov/odep
Provides technical assistance and
information for individuals who have
disabilities.

www.jobaccess.org
A website where people who have
disabilities can post their résumés
and connect with employers to find
jobs.

### Youth Organizations

These organizations welcome all young
people, whether or not they have
physical disabilities. Find listings in
your local phone directory or in your
school or community.

4-H Clubs
Boy Scouts of America
Girl Scouts of America
YMCA
YWCA

# Notes

------------------------------------------------------------------------

### Introduction: Raising Children—Resilient and Ready for Adulthood

p. 6: Christopher Nolan's experience of feeling the cold stream on his feet was described in his book *Under the Eye of the Clock: The Life Story of Christopher Nolan* (New York: St. Martin's Press, 1987).

### Two: Coming Home

p. 57: The different styles that parents use in working with their children's health care teams are described in Susan A. Snell and Karen H. Rosen, "Parents of Special Needs Children Mastering the Job of Parenting," *Contemporary Family Therapy* 19, no. 3 (1997): 425–42.

### Three: Inclusive Parenting: Make It Work for You

p. 97: Beatrice Wright was a pioneer in the study of the psychological experience of living with a physical disability. In *Physical Disability: A Psychosocial Approach* (2nd ed.; New York: Harper and Row, 1983), now a classic in the field, she said that the development of positive self-concept in a person who has a physical disability comes through changes in their values.

### Four: Brothers and Sisters: Siblings Sharing Family Life with Physical Disability in the Mix

p. 106: Twenty-one research studies on the psychological impact of physical disability on siblings were reviewed in Angela Dew, Susan Balandin, and Gwynnyth Llewellyn, "The Psychosocial Impact on Siblings of People with Lifelong Physical Disability: A Review of the Literature," *Journal of Developmental and Physical Disability* 20 (2008): 485–507. The authors concluded that siblings of people who have physical disabilities are mainly positive about their experience, and that there is little difference between siblings who have and who do not have a brother or sister who has a physical disability. They were able to identify only two studies that included the perspectives of the siblings who had the disability and recommend that their input be included in future studies.

p. 107: Parents' attitudes toward their child who has a physical disability is an important factor in sibling adaptation, as discussed in Ineke M. Pit-Ten Cate and

G. M. P. (Ineke) Loots, "Experiences of Siblings of Children with Physical Disabilities: An Empirical Investigation," *Disability and Rehabilitation* 22, no. 9 (2000): 399–408.

p. 120: The finding that physical disability of a sibling was discussed less frequently with his able-bodied siblings than other everyday topics was reported in Ineke M. Pit-Ten Cate and G. M. P. (Ineke) Loots, "Experiences of Siblings of Children with Physical Disabilities: An Empirical Investigation," *Disability and Rehabilitation* 22, no. 9 (2000): 399–408.

p. 124: The Sibshop model of sibling support was developed by Donald Meyer in Seattle, Washington. Sally Conway, in the UK, adapted the program for siblings of children who have developmental disabilities and attend a residential treatment program. The model is described in Sally Conway and Donald Meyer, "Developing Support for Siblings of Young People with Disabilities," *Support for Learning* 23, no. 3 (2008): 113–17.

p. 125: Positive characteristics associated with having a sibling who has a disability are discussed in Paula Dyke, Seonaid Mulroy, and Helen Leonard, "Siblings of Children with Disabilities: Challenges and Opportunities," *Acta Paediatrica* 98 (2009): 23–24.

### Five: Grandparents: Seeing through a New Lens

p. 148: By the time they become grandparents, most people are in the stage of life which Erik Erikson, who proposed a stage theory of adult psychological development, called generativity. At this stage, adults who are beyond child-rearing age continue to be productive in other areas of their lives while also helping the younger generation. Erikson's theory is described in Erik Erikson, *Identity and the Life Cycle* (New York: W. W. Norton, 1994).

### Six: Opening Doors to Inclusion

p. 164: The young woman whose family challenged her to "reach for more" after her spinal cord injury was Kris Ann Piazza, whose story appears in Gary Karp and Stanley D. Klein, eds., *From There to Here: Stories of Adjustment to Spinal Cord Injury* (Horsham, PA: No Limits Communications, 2004), 71.

p. 164: The point that every individual, whether or not he has a physical disability, has some "limitations" that affect his career and avocational options was made by Rhoda Olkin, a psychologist, in her book *What Psychotherapists Should Know about Disability* (New York: Guilford, 1999), 103.

# Index

abortion, 27, 30, 39

academic achievement of child with physical disability, 77, 104, 168; expectations for, 7, 92, 93, 109, 130, 165–66; giving credit for, 98; parents as role models for, 99; pride in, 53. *See also* college attendance; education of child with physical disability

accessibility, 50, 130; advocacy for, 109, 132, 172, 175, 197; home modifications for, 54, 128, 140; ramps for, 47, 54, 128, 140, 195; resources for, 205; in schools/colleges, 52, 109, 132, 176; universal design for, 50, 175, 205

accommodations, 15, 23; advocating for, 197; by employers, 179, 180; at home, 141; at school/college, 38, 63, 171, 176–77, 178

accountability, 7, 167

adjustments: emotional, 50–55; in family life, 14, 47–50; finding your new normal, 68–71, 157

adoption, 10, 11, 29–30, 69, 115; story of family who adopted children with multiple physical disabilities, 155–60

advocacy, xiii, 23, 24, 55, 57, 60, 105, 109, 113, 124, 125, 160, 178, 197–98, 200; for accessibility, 109, 132, 172, 175, 197; for inclusion, 172, 174–75; with insurance company, 66

American Association of Retired Persons, 138, 209

Americans with Disabilities Act (ADA), 63, 180, 208

anger, 24, 31, 35, 48, 54, 76, 129, 190, 198; of child with physical disability, 10, 76, 98, 107; coping with, 84; due to negative stereotypes, 98, 162; of grandparents, 35, 54; of mothers and fathers, 20, 24, 36, 54; rating feelings of, 53; of siblings, xi, 116, 188; at time of diagnosis, 14, 29, 33, 36; toward child with physical disability, 52; toward doctors or medical system, 20, 66, 76; turned into action, 33, 84, 197–98

anxiety: about injury risk, 12–13, 51–52, 94, 95, 103, 164, 168; of child with physical disability, 9, 34; control of, 52, 65; of friends, 31; of grandparents, 54; medications for, 22; of parents, 10, 22, 24, 31, 51, 52, 58, 61, 94, 102, 193; regarding prognosis, 61; related to teen with a new physical disability, 170

appearance and clothing, 11, 173

architectural barriers, 50, 173, 175, 197

arts, 5, 42, 141, 158, 174, 202, 203; resources for, 212–13

attitudes about physical disability, xiii, 50–53, 127, 162–63, 201, 215n; adjustment of, 14, 40; "altitude of attitude," 163; as barriers, 173, 184; bullying, 173; negative, 13, 15, 44, 50, 51, 52–53, 98, 101, 162–63; parental modeling of, 99, 163; person-centered, 158; positive, 37, 51, 52, 69, 80, 99, 103, 107, 163

handicapped parking spaces, 189, 197
head injury, 59
health insurance, 21, 23, 37, 62, 83;
    COBRA, 21; lack or inadequacy of, xi,
    82, 83, 144; learning about benefits
    from, 63; managing problems with,
    21, 65–66; Medicaid, 42, 209; services
    that may not be covered by, 63, 67,
    127; social workers' help with, 66
help from others: balancing self-
    sufficiency with, 196–97; financial (*see*
    financial assistance); peer support and
    education, 67–68; for problem solving,
    55, 90, 169; professional help for emo-
    tional reactions, 54, 55; for respite care,
    81; between siblings, 114–19, 168, 189;
    teaching child to ask for, 169–70
helplessness, 32; of fathers, 22, 32; vs.
    rewards of parenting, 99; at time of
    diagnosis, 14, 27, 32, 128; turned to
    action, 37–38, 197
hobbies: of child with physical disability,
    98, 164, 165, 166, 171; of grandparents,
    150; of parents, 16, 85, 199, 200–201
home care services, 81–82, 155–56
homecoming from the hospital, 46–71,
    128; becoming an expert on your
    child's physical disability, 62–68, 102;
    emotional adjustments to, 50–55; fam-
    ily life adjustments to, 47–50; finding
    your new normal, 68–71, 157; medical
    care and, 56–62
home modifications, 54, 128, 140;
    resources for, 205
homeschooling, 158, 176
hope, 55; of grandparents, 55, 148, 149,
    199; loss of, at time of diagnosis, 28;
    spirituality and, 38, 39, 190; of teens
    with a physical disability, 184
horseback riding, 5, 6, 13, 49, 97, 145,
    174, 190, 198, 212
hospitalizations, xi, 12, 51, 91, 113, 129,
    141
hot-weather activities, 22
humor/laughter: to diffuse conflicts, 111;
    in family, 41, 43, 44–45, 83, 91, 111,
    203; parental modeling of, 83, 99; of
    person with physical disability, 11, 97,
    188; between siblings, 110
hydrocephalus, 28, 30, 128

inclusive parenting, ix–xiii, 1–2, 16, 14,
    79–101; building a resilient family,
    1–16, 79, 90–99; coping with emo-
    tions, 84–85; creating your unique
    family, 100; finding your new normal,
    68–71, 157; getting support for,
    79–84; reaping rewards of, 99–100;
    taking care of yourself, 85–90, 104–5,
    202; tips for, 101
independence, preparing child for, 4–13,
    15, 92–99, 101, 161–85, 216n; allow-
    ing risk taking, 11–13, 43–44, 52, 78,
    94–96, 101, 116, 168–69, 189; balanc-
    ing dreams and limitations, 164–66,
    179–80; combating stereotypes and
    negative attitudes, 162–63; communi-
    cating confidence in child, 163–64;
    determining needed resources, 171; in
    education, 176–78; expecting success,
    x–xi, 2, 3, 92–93, 108–9; experiences,
    4–7; laying the groundwork, 162–71;
    making a plan, 171–85; managing
    medical and physical care, 180–83;
    next steps for parents, 185; providing
    positive role models, 96–99, 162, 163,
    166; sexuality, dating, and marriage,
    15, 171, 183–85; social life and recre-
    ation, 9–11, 77–78, 101, 172–76;
    teaching child to ask for help, 169–70;
    teaching responsibility, 7–9, 93–94,
    101, 108–11, 166–68; teen with a new
    disability, 170–71; vocational training
    and employment, 15, 66, 158, 178–80
Individualized Educational Plan (IEP),
    177
Individuals with Disabilities Education
    Act, 176
injuries, anxiety about, 12–13, 51–52,
    94, 95, 103, 164, 168. *See also* frac-
    tures in osteogenesis imperfecta; safety
intellectual ability of child, 70, 156, 158,
    171; recognition and valuing of, 70,
    97, 164, 165, 180, 190
intellectual activities, 5, 123, 164, 165
intellectual closeness between grand-
    parents and child, 145, 157
intellectual disability, 63, 116
intellectually gifted child, 157, 164
Internet, 34, 37, 38, 62, 63, 84, 137,
    172

intimate relationships: of parents, 80–81, 101, 140, 201; of young adults with physical disabilities, 15, 172, 183–84
isolation, 53, 121, 160

jealousy of siblings, 46, 107, 109, 110, 111–12, 116, 129
jobs. *See* employment
journaling, 36–37, 53

laughter. *See* humor/laughter
learning: about your child's physical disability, 28, 37, 42, 62–68, 102; about health insurance, 63; from other parents, 89–90
least restrictive environment, 63, 176
legal protections, 63, 172, 176, 180, 208, 209
leg braces, x, xi, 5, 7, 12, 13, 47, 87, 96, 97, 129, 184
leukemia-related paralysis, story of family who has child with, 75–78
living independently, 171, 181, 193. *See also* independence, preparing child for
loneliness, 14, 32, 34
looking ahead to what you want, 199–203
loss, feelings of: after children leave home, 192, 197; of grandparents, 54, 147; of parents, 28, 33, 50, 76, 160; related to teen with a new physical disability, 170; due to separation from child, 33, 34; at time of diagnosis, 29, 35

marriage: of parents, 80–81; preparing teens with physical disabilities for, 15, 171, 183–85; resources for, 207
Medicaid, 42, 209
medical care, 2, 13, 56–62; adoption of children with significant physical disabilities, 155–58; communication with medical team about, 57–61; getting answers to your questions about, 61–62, 159; grandparents' role in, 64–65; including child in decisions about, 62, 181–82; partnering with professionals for, 65–67, 101; peer support and education about, 67–68; teaching teens to manage, 180–83. *See*

*also* doctors/medical team; hospitalizations; surgeries
mental health care, 3, 54, 55, 66–67, 93, 97, 101, 196; resources for, 209–10
multigenerational families, 101, 135–37, 193
muscular dystrophy, 55, 142, 147
music activities, x, 5, 12, 86, 94, 104, 141, 144, 167, 174, 188, 189

neonatal intensive care unit, 19–21
new normal for your family, 68–71, 157
news of child's physical disability, 26–40; grandparents' emotional reactions to, 20, 34–35; parents' initial emotional reactions to, 14, 19–20, 31–33; receiving after birth or later in childhood, 28–30, 41, 187; receiving before birth, 26–28, 33, 102, 127–28; ripple effects of, 30–31; separation from child and, 33–34; ways of coping with, 35–39
Nolan, Christopher, 6, 215n
nurses, 21, 28, 34, 58, 101, 186; cost of hiring, 157, 193; for respite care, 82

Olkin, Rhoda, 161, 165, 216n
optimism: of grandparents, 148, 149; of parents, 28, 29. *See also* hope
osteogenesis imperfecta (OI): advocacy and fund raising for, 105, 148, 203; fracture risk in, 12, 13, 41, 43, 56, 62, 70, 92, 96, 99, 102–4, 110, 113, 168, 181, 182; grandparents of child with, 54–55, 105, 139, 148; medical care for, 42, 62, 64, 181, 183, 193; misinformation given to parents about, 41, 58–59; negative attitudes about, 44; online support group for, 42; parents educating doctors about, 64, 102; parent self-care and, 85; parents learning about, 28, 37, 42, 62, 64, 102; preparing young adult for independence, 161, 164, 174, 180–83; psychotherapy for person with, 66–67; receiving diagnosis of, 28–29, 41, 102; resources for, 207, 210; risk taking and, 13, 95, 96–97; safety concerns for child with, 49, 52, 70, 91, 95, 97, 108, 181; siblings of child with, 70, 104, 113–14, 117, 121;

single parent of child with, 83, 196; socialization of child with, 174; sports participation and, 13, 91, 108; stories of families who have a child with, 41–45, 102–5; young adults with, 193

Osteogenesis Imperfecta Foundation (OIF), xiii, 64, 203, 210

paraplegia, 1, 76, 165, 170, 180, 184, 185. *See also* spinal cord injury

para-transit system, 175

parents: balancing self-sufficiency with help from others, 196–97; becoming experts on your child's physical disability, 28, 37, 42, 62–68, 102; building resilient families, 1–16, 79, 90–99 (*see also* resilient families); as case managers, 22–23, 63, 64, 155; divorce of, 1, 33, 43, 67, 83, 115, 117, 119, 196, 203; emotional reactions to news of child's physical disability, 14, 19–20, 31–33; employment of, 20, 21, 33, 48, 77, 79, 83, 87, 117, 155–56, 196, 200; empty nesters, 15–16, 196, 200, 204; friendships of, 23, 30–31, 32, 35, 38, 42, 48–49, 50, 54, 79, 82–86, 88–89, 201; grandparents functioning as, 142–43; hobbies and interests of, 16, 85, 199, 200–201; inclusive, 14, 79–101 (*see also* inclusive parenting); intimacy between, 80–81; learning from other parents, 89–90; looking ahead to what you want, 199–203; meeting each child's needs, 2, 24–25, 90–92, 103, 107–8, 189–90; moving forward, 203–4; patience and tolerance of, 15, 78, 98, 100, 167, 194, 198–99; peer support and education for, 67–68; personal growth of, 190–91, 194–99; positive role modeling by, 96–99, 162, 163; preparing child for independence, 161–85; protectiveness of, 12, 52, 95, 96, 99, 102–5, 109, 119, 168, 170; pursuing your passions, 202–3; rebuilding your social life, 201–2; reconnecting with spouse or partner, 201; resources for, 205–13; retirement of, 12, 16, 30, 144, 150, 200; self-confidence of, 3, 15, 39, 56,

59, 95, 101, 139, 185, 194–95, 196, 203; siblings functioning as, 116–17, 118–19; single, 21, 35, 47, 48, 49, 82–84, 85, 87, 155, 196, 199, 201, 202; support for, 14, 79–84; taking care of yourself, 85–90, 104–5, 202; teamwork of, 80, 102–4, 159; thankfulness of, 77, 129, 192, 194; time management for, 14, 47–48, 86–88; trusting your instincts, 13, 15, 58, 60, 195; turning anger into action, 197–98; volunteer work of, 49, 86, 200, 203; who have a physical disability, 99, 206

parking in handicapped spaces, 189, 197

parties, birthday, 158, 173

pastoral counselors, 55

patience: of grandparents, 148, 199; of parents, 15, 78, 98, 100, 167, 194, 198–99; of siblings, 107, 113, 125, 157

pediatric intensive care unit, 38

peer support and education, 67–68

personal care attendant (PCA), 109, 131, 171, 177, 178, 181

personal growth of parents, 190–91, 194–99

physical therapists, 101, 177

physical therapy, x, xi, 6, 82, 116, 122, 142, 187

physicians. *See* doctors/medical team

polio, x–xi, 26, 53, 69, 112, 114, 164, 169

positive expectations, x–xi, 2, 3, 92–93, 108–9

positive role models, 96–99, 162, 163, 166

postconcussive syndrome, 59

pragmatism, 3

prejudices, 52, 77, 121, 197. *See also* attitudes about physical disability; stereotypes

premature birth, 155, 186, 198

pride: of child with physical disability, 13, 83; of grandparents, 104; of parents, xi, 30, 53, 83, 95, 192; of siblings, 115, 116, 125, 129

priority setting: grandparents' role and, 141, 148; to meet family needs, 90, 94; to meet immediate needs of child with physical disability, 2, 87, 91; to meet parents' time and energy needs, 47, 79, 87, 194, 202

166, 167, 169, 193; of grandparents, 149; of parents, 3, 15, 39, 56, 59, 95, 101, 139, 185, 194–95, 196, 203

self-esteem: building in child, 4, 52, 53, 96–99, 164; parent role modeling of, 79, 96; of parents, 88, 139

sex education, 184

sexual abuse or exploitation, 184

sexuality: of parents, 80–81; resources for, 207; of young adults with physical disabilities, 15, 171, 183–85

sexually transmitted diseases, 184

shyness, 9, 10, 12, 58, 70

siblings, 14–15, 103, 106–26, 187–91, 215–16n; age differences between, 114; assigning chores to, x, 6, 7–8, 44, 46, 47, 83, 87, 93–94, 104, 109–11, 161, 167, 168, 171, 189; babysitting by, 111, 117, 120, 168; in blended families, 43, 156, 157; communication by, 112–13, 120; "cope-ability" for, 15, 119–24; friends of, 123–24; growing together, 124–26; helping each other, 114–19, 168, 189; jealousy, guilt and rivalry among, 46, 91, 107, 109, 110, 111–12, 116, 129; meeting each child's needs, 2, 24–25, 90–92, 103, 107–8, 189–90; in parental role, 116–17, 118–19; parents setting the stage for relationships between, 107–11; reframing who you are, 122–23; spirituality of, 121–22; support groups for, 124; view of disabilities, 69–71, 124–27

Sibshop model of sibling support, 124, 212, 216n

single parents: self-care of, 85, 202; social life of, 201; support for, 35, 48, 49, 82–84, 196; time and energy demands on, 47, 87

Skype, 137

social life: of child with physical disability, ix, xi, xii, 9–11, 44, 77–78, 101, 115, 171, 172–76; of parents after children leave home, 199, 201–2, 203; of siblings, 117. See also friendships

social support, 38, 48–49, 63, 126, 146

social workers, 42, 55, 66, 67, 101, 155, 210

spasticity, 145, 157, 160

speech problems, 155, 156, 157

spina bifida (SB), 1, 99, 195, 196; balancing dreams and limitations of child with, 165; college attendance for young adult with, 178, 193; demands of caring for child with, 46, 47, 91; expectations for child with, 109, 167; grandparents of child with, 81, 135, 139, 144; receiving diagnosis of, 27–29, 30, 33, 84; resources for, 207, 208; rewards of parenting a child with, 79; sexuality, dating, marriage and, 183; siblings of child with, 116, 118, 127, 129; sports participation and, 6–7; story of family who has child with, 127–32; support group for, 68; travel for child with, 91

Spina Bifida Association, xiii, 128, 210

spinal cord injury (SCI), xii, xiii, 83; due to birth injury, 19–20; due to car crash, 55, 59, 60, 143, 170, 178; encouraging abilities of child with, 96, 98, 163–64; family priority setting related to, 87; leukemia-related, 75–78, 80, 99; resources for, 207, 208, 210; single parent of child with, 83; stories of families who have a child with, 19–25, 75–78; in young adults, 119, 170. See also paraplegia; quadriplegia

spirituality and religious beliefs, 162; anger/questioning God, 23, 32, 38; of grandparents, 54, 131, 143, 147; homeschooling and, 176; lack of, 39; of siblings, 121, 190; strength and comfort provided by, 39, 76, 82, 84, 131, 159, 190

"spoiled" children, 93, 109, 167

sports activities, 1, 2, 5, 49, 67, 75, 98, 104, 113, 130, 134, 165, 171, 174–75, 188, 189, 190; adaptive, 6, 7, 78, 97, 175; for child with osteogenesis imperfecta, 13, 91, 108; for child with spina bifida, 6–7; resources for, 211–12; risk taking and, 11–13, 43–44, 52, 78, 94–96, 168; on special-needs teams, 23; for wheelchair athletes, 75, 77–78, 94–95, 166, 173

stereotypes, 15, 29, 52, 68, 98, 100, 101, 123, 162, 166, 183